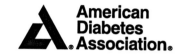

American
Diabetes
Association.

MEETING THE
AMERICAN
DIABETES
ASSOCIATION
STANDARDS
OF CARE   SECOND
EDITION

An Algorithmic Approach
to Clinical Care of
the Diabetes Patient

T0179694

Mayer B. Davidson, MD, and Stanley H. Hsia, MD

Director, Book Publishing, Abe Ogden; *Managing Editor*, Rebekah Renshaw; *Acquisitions Editor*, Victor Van Beuren; *Editor*, Wendy M. Martin-Shuma; *Production Manager and Composition*, Melissa Sprott; *Printer*, Lightning Source.

Printed in the United States of America
1 3 5 7 9 10 8 6 4 2

The suggestions and information contained in this publication are generally consistent with the *Standards of Medical Care in Diabetes* and other policies of the American Diabetes Association, but they do not represent the policy or position of the Association or any of its boards or committees. Reasonable steps have been taken to ensure the accuracy of the information presented. However, the American Diabetes Association cannot ensure the safety or efficacy of any product or service described in this publication. Individuals are advised to consult a physician or other appropriate health care professional before undertaking any diet or exercise program or taking any medication referred to in this publication. Professionals must use and apply their own professional judgment, experience, and training and should not rely solely on the information contained in this publication before prescribing any diet, exercise, or medication. The American Diabetes Association—its officers, directors, employees, volunteers, and members—assumes no responsibility or liability for personal or other injury, loss, or damage that may result from the suggestions or information in this publication.

⊗ The paper in this publication meets the requirements of the ANSI Standard Z39.48-1992 (permanence of paper).

ADA titles may be purchased for business or promotional use or for special sales. To purchase more than 50 copies of this book at a discount, or for custom editions of this book with your logo, contact the American Diabetes Association at the address below or at booksales@diabetes.org.

American Diabetes Association
2451 Crystal Drive, Suite 900
Arlington, VA 22202

Library of Congress Cataloging-in-Publication Data
Names: Davidson, Mayer B., author. | Hsia, Stanley H., author. | American Diabetes Association, issuing body.
Title: Meeting the American Diabetes Association standards of care / Mayer B. Davidson and Stanley H. Hsia.
Description: 2nd edition. | Alexandria : American Diabetes Association, [2017] | Includes bibliographical references and index.
Identifiers: LCCN 2016041977 | ISBN 9781580406017
Subjects: | MESH: Diabetes Mellitus--therapy | Clinical Protocols--standards | Reference Standards | United States
Classification: LCC RC660 | NLM WK 815 | DDC 362.1964/6200973--dc23
LC record available at https://lccn.loc.gov/2016041977

This book is dedicated to the following midlevel providers in appreciation for their successful efforts to improve diabetes outcomes in the patients under their care:

Katherine Arce, NP ∎ Katie Asmuth, NP
Wanda Butts, NP ∎ Susan Campos, NP
Diana Cano, PA ∎ Maria Blanco-Castellanos, RN
Antoinette Chavez, RN ∎ Lenore Coleman, PharmD
Mary Rose Deraco, RN ∎ Tamara Douglas, RN
Cynthia Dunlop, RN ∎ Lisa Flynn, PA
Simi Gandhi, NP ∎ Bart Gilliam, PA
Joyce Ivy, NP ∎ LaKesha Johnson, PA
Guy Keppler, NP ∎ Lisa Kirchen, RN
Gina Lau, PharmD ∎ Alex Le, PA
Arlene Lopez-Glass, PA ∎ Teresa Luna, RN
Evelin Martinez, PA ∎ Apollonia Mendoza, NP
Nilda Molina, Pharm D ∎ Freddy Montenegro, NP
Maria Navar, NP ∎ Mary Pearce, NP ∎ Levi Ramos, NP
Latoya Reinhold, NP ∎ Beverly Rockwell, RN
Kristina Romero, NP ∎ Manuela Romo, RN
Carol Rosenburg, RN ∎ Ligaya Scarlett, NP
Dilcia Sealey, NP ∎ Elizabeth Spinella, NP
Thelma Staples, NP ∎ Christine Turner, PA
Alana Wilson, RN ∎ Barbara Wisehart, NP

and any others whom I might have inadvertently missed.

Contents

Preface

During the senior author's training in the 1960s, the prevailing opinion was that diabetes control did not affect its complications; they were genetically determined. Thus, clinically, we were taught that our goal was simply to keep the patient asymptomatic. In the 1970s, enough animal and observational data became available to convince some of us that diabetes control was extremely important to forestall the microvascular complications.[1] Battles raged between the minority who believed that attaining near-euglycemia was beneficial and the majority who favored the genetic hypothesis. It was not until the publication in 1993 of the Diabetes Control and Complications Trial, evaluating patients with type 1 diabetes, that the importance of diabetes control for microvascular complications was finally accepted.[2] The publication of the UK Prospective Diabetes Study (UKPDS) in 1998 confirmed this conclusion in people with type 2 diabetes as well.[3] In parallel, evidence became available that control of blood pressure (BP)[4] and LDL cholesterol[5] levels was also critically important to forestall the macrovascular complications.

The challenge for providers caring for people with diabetes is how to achieve the glycemic, BP, and LDL cholesterol goals. The number of possible medications to use is large. For instance, there are 11 classes of non-insulin drugs to treat hyperglycemia (see Chapter 3, Table 3.1) with a number of drugs in each class and over 20 different insulin preparations. When and how to use these drugs can be quite perplexing. It is our hope that the information in this volume will clarify these issues for the reader. We know that the algorithms described in this book can be effective. For example, a registered nurse (not a nurse practitioner) trained in the use of the algorithms was placed in a family medicine clinic under the supervision of the primary care physicians, who referred 178 out-of-control patients to her, 111 of whom were already taking insulin. After 9–12 months, the mean baseline A1C level of 11.1% in these 178 patients was lowered to 7.2%, with 49% meeting the American Diabetes Association goal of <7.0%. Furthermore, 90% met the BP goal of <130/80 mmHg, and 96% met the LDL cholesterol goal of <100 mg/dL.[6] Thus, we have no doubt that if these algorithms for non-pregnant adults are followed, glycemic, lipid, and BP outcome measures will improve considerably, which will result in significantly less microvascular and macrovascular complications in people with diabetes.

Although other states may have different requirements, in California, nurse practitioners can practice independently, physician assistants must practice under the supervision of a physician and other midlevel providers (e.g., registered nurses), and clinical pharmacists may follow protocols approved by the institution or organization in which they work. The authors do not know the regulations regarding midlevel providers in other countries.

REFERENCES

1. Davidson M. The case for control in diabetes mellitus. *West J Med* 1978;129:193–200

2. Diabetes Control and Complications Trial Research Group. The effect of intensive treatment of diabetes on the development and progression of long-term complications in insulin-independent diabetes mellitus. *N Engl J Med* 1993;329:977–986

3. UK Prospective Diabetes Study Group. Intensive blood-glucose control with sulphonylureas or insulin compared with conventional treatment and risk of complications in patients with type 2 diabetes (UKPDS 33). *Lancet* 1998;352:837–853

4. Emdin CA, Rahimi K, Neal B, et al. Blood pressure lowering in type 2 diabetes: a systematic review and meta-analysis. *JAMA* 2015;313:603–615

5. Cholesterol Treatment Trialists' Collaborators. Efficacy and safety of cholesterol-lowering treatment: prospective meta-analysis of data from 90,056 participants in 14 randomized trials of statins. *Lancet* 2005;366:1267–1278

6. Davidson MB, Blanco-Castellanos M, Duran P. Integrating nurse-directed diabetes management into a primary care setting. *Am J Manag Care* 2010;16:652–656

Acknowledgments

I wish to acknowledge two people who were instrumental (for different reasons) for my success with detailed treatment algorithms to improve diabetes care. Thirty-three years ago, Richard C. Ossorio, MD, the Medical Director of the Cedars-Sinai HMO, curbed the high cost of HIV disease by directing patients to several infectious disease specialists who developed a protocol for their care. After this success, Dr. Ossorio approached me to develop a program for the care of diabetic patients, and nurse-directed care was born. Writing detailed treatment algorithms was one of the most challenging intellectual exercises I've undertaken. In these algorithms, there can be no "clinical judgments"; there has to be a specific instruction for the midlevel provider depending on specific individual circumstances (i.e., the dose of the medications in response to the laboratory or self-monitored blood glucose results, LDL cholesterol concentrations, or blood pressure). Only when the circumstances fall outside of the treatment algorithms should the supervisory physician be called. For greatest efficiency, this interaction needs to be infrequent. Anne L. Peters, MD, my fellow at the time Dr. Ossorio approached me, has a marvelously logical mind and was extremely helpful in compiling the original and early renditions of the treatment algorithms. I am grateful to both of them for starting me on this 33-year quest to improve diabetes care.

—*Mayer B. Davidson, MD*

Chapter 1
Laying the Groundwork

BACKGROUND FOR EVIDENCE-BASED ADA GUIDELINES FOR STANDARDS OF DIABETES CARE

Diabetes has a profound effect on the health of our population and, in 2012, imposed an estimated cost to the U.S. health care system of $245 billion.[1] Diabetic retinopathy is the leading cause of new cases of blindness in people between the ages of 20 and 74 years in developed countries.[2] Diabetic kidney disease is the leading cause of patients with end-stage renal disease.[3] Diabetic peripheral neuropathy is an underlying cause of nontraumatic lower-extremity amputations in diabetic patients.[4] More than half of lower-extremity amputations, and in some populations up to 90%, occur in people with diabetes.[5] The prevalence of coronary artery disease is twofold higher in men with diabetes and fourfold higher in women with diabetes, compared with appropriate nondiabetic control subjects.[6] Strokes are two to three times more common in people with diabetes than in people without the disease.[7] Peripheral arterial disease is also much more common in diabetic patients than in nondiabetic individuals.[8] Even as complication rates have declined over the past 20 years, rates of myocardial infarctions, strokes, amputations, and end-stage renal disease remain substantially higher in people with diabetes than in those without diabetes.[9]

Much of this devastation can be avoided. The microvascular complications of diabetes could be markedly reduced, if not eliminated, if blood glucose targets are achieved. Progression of early kidney disease to late-stage nephropathy can be forestalled by appropriate (nonglycemic) therapy. Although macrovascular disease cannot be entirely prevented, its effects can be sharply curtailed with appropriate treatment for lipids and blood pressure (BP), smoking cessation, and ingestion of aspirin. Evidence for these important assertions will be briefly summarized.

GLYCEMIA

There have been five prospective studies in over 2,000 type 1[10–12] and type 2[13,14] diabetic patients demonstrating that there is virtually no development or progression of retinopathy and nephropathy over 4–9 years if mean hemoglobin A_{1c} (A1C) levels are maintained at <7.0%. Intervention studies have also demonstrated that more intensive lowering of hyperglycemia results in substantially less microvascular complications, proving a causative relationship between improved glycemic control and these improved outcomes. For type 1 diabetic patients, the landmark Diabetes Control and Complications Trial (DCCT) showed that intensive glycemic control that achieved a mean A1C level of ~7% dramatically reduced the development and progression of retinopathy, albuminuria, and clinical neuropathy as compared to conventional therapy that remained at an A1C of ~9%.[15] Even years after the DCCT ended, when the between-group difference in glycemic control had virtually disappeared, the Epidemiology of Diabetes Interventions and Complications (EDIC) long-term follow-up found that the formerly intensively controlled patients still had less retinopathy, albuminuria, and neuropathy symptoms compared to the formerly conventionally treated patients who had intensified their control only after the study had ended.[16-20] These data demonstrate the long-term durability of the microvascular benefits of intensive glycemic control and therefore the enduring value of early intensive treatment. For type 2 diabetic patients, the Kumamoto Study showed that more intensive control with multiple daily insulin injections substantially reduced progression of retinopathy, nephropathy, and nerve conduction impairment.[13] The landmark UK Prospective Diabetes Study (UKPDS) showed that intensive glycemic control with either oral agents or insulin that achieved a mean A1C of 7.0% significantly reduced microvascular end points as compared to conventional treatment that achieved an A1C of only 7.9%.[21] And similar to the EDIC findings, long-term follow-up of the UKPDS patients, even after the between-group difference in glycemic control had disappeared, showed that microvascular complications remained significantly less among patients who were formerly intensively treated.[22] These data demonstrate the durability of the protection against progression of microvascular complications and thus the value of early intensive treatment in type 2 diabetes as well.

More recently, three additional trials targeting A1C levels below 7.0% demonstrated some further reduction of microvascular outcomes, albeit to a lesser absolute benefit given that the curvilinear relationship between glycemia and microvascular complications reflects smaller absolute changes at lower A1C levels (as represented in Figure 1.1). In the Action to Control Cardiovascular Risk in Diabetes (ACCORD) trial, intensive treatment that achieved a nadir A1C level of 6.3%, as compared to 7.6% in the standard control group, still produced a 21% and 31% relative reduction in incident micro- and macroalbuminuria, respectively, along with significant improvements in a few peripheral neuropathy measures.[23] Even after 8 years of follow-up, prior intensive glucose control still had a lasting effect to reduce retinopathy progression.[24] In the Action in Diabetes and Vascular Disease: Preterax and Diamicron Modified Release Controlled Evaluation (ADVANCE) study, which achieved an A1C level of 6.5% with intensive treatment compared to standard treatment, which only achieved a 7.3% level, there was still a 21% reduction in the incidence of nephropathy.[25] However, the Veterans Affairs Diabetes Trial (VADT), in which intensive treatment achieved an A1C of 6.9% compared to 8.4% in the standard therapy group, failed to show further reductions in microvascular outcomes.[26] These latter studies therefore show that further reduction of A1C below 7.0% may still produce additional microvascular benefits (principally reduced albuminuria), albeit less profoundly and consistently than compared to A1C lowering from higher baseline levels. However, in all instances for both type 1 and type 2 diabetes, intensive control down to lower A1C levels entails a substantially greater incidence of symptomatic

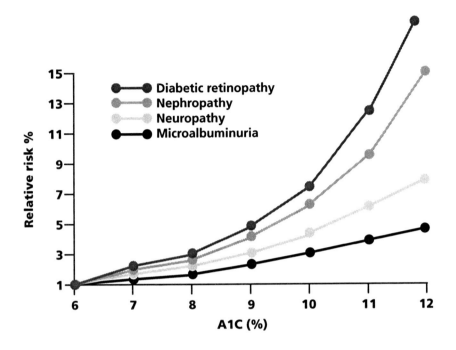

Figure 1.1. Relative risk of progression of diabetic complications, by mean A1C level (based on DCCT data[10]).

hypoglycemia,[15,21,25-27] which will not only limit the extent to which "near-normal" glycemic control can be achieved, but may entail increased risks that could offset the progressively diminishing microvascular benefits as tighter control is pursued.

As for the macrovascular complications of diabetes, the data are much weaker, at least in the shorter term, but longer-term data do support some measurable benefit of achieving tighter glycemic control. Earlier prospective cohort studies showed that the direct association between hyperglycemia and atherosclerotic cardiovascular disease (ASCVD) extends all the way down into the mid-normal range. For instance, in the EPIC-Norfolk cohort of men age 45–79 years, the 4-year rate of ischemic heart disease was 2.7-fold higher in those with A1C levels of 5.0–5.4% as compared to those with A1C <5.0%.[28] In the Atherosclerosis Risk in Communities (ARIC) cohort, among nondiabetic adults, every 1% increase in A1C was associated with a 2.4-fold higher relative risk for ASCVD over 8–10 years, a relationship that extended down to an A1C level as low as 4.6%.[29] One meta-analysis of glucose-lowering interventions in comparison to conventional treatment that included 1,800 type 1 and 4,472 type 2 diabetic patients found substantial macrovascular event reductions with interventions to improve glucose control compared to conventional treatment, in both groups of diabetic patients and particularly among younger patients with shorter diabetes duration.[30]

Although the original DCCT in type 1 diabetic patients showed a 41% reduction in macrovascular events that was not statistically significant, a further 9-year follow-up of the EDIC cohort eventually showed a significant 42% reduction in ASCVD events in individuals who were originally treated intensively compared to those treated conventionally.[31] Even after more than 30 years of cumulative observation, the lower risk of both micro- and macrovascular complications associated with original intensive treatment has remained significant,[32,33] and even all-cause mortality was significantly reduced.[34] Similarly, among type 2 diabetic patients, although the original UKPDS showed a 16% reduction in ASCVD events that just missed statistical significance, just as with the data in type 1 diabetes, after a further 10 years of follow-up, a significant 15% reduction in myocardial infarctions (MIs) and a significant 13% reduction in all-cause mortality emerged, despite the convergence of the original difference in glycemic control between groups.[22]

The more recent ACCORD, ADVANCE, and VADT studies were actually specifically designed to examine macrovascular outcomes, but so far, their findings in this regard have been less favorable. In ACCORD, 35% of the 10,251 subjects had a previous ASCVD event at baseline, and after 3.5 years of follow-up, not only was the primary outcome of composite ASCVD events not significantly lower with intensive treatment, but the study was stopped prematurely because of a significantly *higher* ASCVD and all-cause mortality in the intensively treated group (achieving a median A1C of 6.4%) compared with the control group (achieving a median A1C of 7.5%), despite a significantly lower rate of nonfatal MIs.[27] Follow-up reports 5 and 9 years after study termination still showed persistence of the higher mortality rate from intensive treatment.[35,36] As yet, there is no good explanation for this unexpected observation; increased episodes of severe hypoglycemia did not adequately account for the higher mortality, and many other confounding factors complicated the analyses.[37] In ADVANCE, 32% of the 11,140 patients had a history of major macrovascular disease at baseline, and after 5 years of follow-up, effects on major macrovascular events failed to reach statistical significance with intensive control compared to standard treatment.[25] In the VADT, 40% of the 1,791 veterans had a prior ASCVD event at baseline, and after 5.6 years of follow-up, there was no significant difference in any major ASCVD events in the intensively treated group compared to the standard treatment group.[26] A subsequent meta-analysis of combined data from the UKPDS, ACCORD, ADVANCE, and VADT found a significant 9% reduction in major ASCVD events (including a 15% reduction in MIs) but found no reductions in mortality; yet there were significantly greater hypoglycemic events.[38]

Based on the foregoing body of data, the American Diabetes Association (ADA) currently recommends a general A1C treatment goal of ≤7.0% for all nonpregnant diabetic adults[39] to reduce microvascular complications, particularly if implemented soon after the diagnosis of diabetes, which may be associated with long-term macrovascular risk reduction as well. However, a more stringent A1C target (e.g., <6.5%) may be reasonable for some individuals who can still avoid hypoglycemia, such as patients with shorter duration of diabetes, no significant ASCVD history, and/or longer life expectancy. Conversely, a less stringent A1C target may be more appropriate for those patients who have significant comorbidities or advanced complications, limited life expectancy, or substantial risk of severe hypoglycemia or if the general goal of ≤7.0% cannot be easily achieved without hypoglycemia despite appropriate education, monitoring, and treatment. Individualized clinical judgment should be used to determine the appropriate A1C goal in each case, based on each patient's needs, preferences, and values.

DYSLIPIDEMIA

There is a strong body of evidence showing that HMG-CoA reductase inhibitors (statins) effectively reduce nonfatal ASCVD events (both MIs and strokes), ASCVD deaths, and total mortality in the general population.[40] Also, more intensive statin therapy reduces more ASCVD events than less intensive therapy.[41] In patients with diabetes, the relative risk reduction is the same as for nondiabetic individuals[40-42] (although the data are much weaker for individuals with type 1 diabetes[41,42]). However, the absolute risk reduction is threefold greater in diabetic patients[43] because of the higher baseline absolute risk of diabetic patients compared to individuals without diabetes. A meta-analysis of statin trials involving diabetic patients also showed that the relative risk reduction of statin use is similar irrespective of baseline levels of LDL cholesterol or BMI in older versus younger diabetic patients, in men versus women, and in individuals with or without existing vascular disease.[42] Over 4.3 years of follow-up, for every ~40 mg/dL (1 mmol/L) fall in LDL cholesterol, there is a 9% relative reduction in all-cause mortality and a 20–25% relative reduction in major coronary or vascular events, strokes, or the need for revascularization.[42] Among studies of diabetic patients for primary prevention of ASCVD (i.e., no previous ASCVD), statin treatment of 37 individuals over 4.5 years will prevent one major coronary event, whereas in secondary prevention (i.e., previous ASCVD history), statin treatment of only 15 individuals over 5.1 years will prevent one major coronary event.[43] Statin use in diabetes has previously been shown to be cost-effective, even for primary prevention.[44]

The ADA previously recommended that all diabetic patients over age 40 years with at least 1 ASCVD risk factor (family history of ASCVD, smoking, hypertension, dyslipidemia, or albuminuria) should receive a statin regardless of their baseline LDL cholesterol level and that statins should also be considered for younger or lower-risk patients if their LDL cholesterol level was above target (<100 mg/dL for patients without clinical evidence of ASCVD or <70 mg/dL for patients with clinical evidence of ASCVD).[45] These recommendations were largely consistent with the National Cholesterol Education Program's Third Adult Treatment Panel (ATP-III) recommendations for the general population.[46,47] However, revised guidelines from the American Heart Association and the American College of Cardiology (AHA/ACC) in 2013 highlighted the lack of randomized controlled trial evidence directly supporting the use of such absolute LDL cholesterol targets in optimally guiding statin use and instead emphasized the proportional reduction (% lowering) of LDL cholesterol by using statin formulations of varying intensities as a more evidence-based treatment strategy.[48] The ADA has since revised its own recommendations for diabetic patients to be more consistent with these AHA/ACC guidelines: a high-intensity statin should be used in patients of any age with overt ASCVD and considered in patients of any age without overt ASCVD but with additional ASCVD risk factors; a moderate-intensity statin should be considered in patients over age 40 years without additional ASCVD risk factors or in patients under age 40 years with additional ASCVD risk factors.[49] However, substantial controversy currently surrounds the AHA/ACC guidelines, since many lipid experts still prefer to apply the ATP-III targets. Decades of accumulated scientific evidence on the role of cholesterol in atherosclerosis show that cholesterol levels correlate directly, independently, and continuously with absolute ASCVD risk, and this evidence is therefore consistent with the general principle, "the lower the cholesterol, the better," with as yet no demonstrable lower limit.[50] Thus, there is concern that by taking the emphasis off the aggressive pursuit of defined cholesterol targets, the AHA/ACC guidelines may not as effectively address the inadequately treated hypercholesterolemia that is still prevalent in the population. For example, before the introduction of the AHA/ACC guidelines, one recent survey showed that, despite improvements over the past 20 years, only 30% of the highest-risk individuals in the U.S. successfully met their ATP-III LDL cholesterol targets.[51]

Recognizing the potential merits of both approaches, our treatment algorithm at this time will follow the current ADA recommendations initially, but if ATP-III targets are not met by that strategy alone, treatment will be further intensified until ATP-III targets are met. If maximum-tolerated doses of a statin are insufficient to achieve LDL cholesterol targets, then addition of a second LDL cholesterol–lowering agent to provide additive effect should be considered (e.g., ezetimibe or bile acid sequestrants). It should be noted that there is as yet limited evidence of additive ASCVD risk reduction using combinations of LDL cholesterol–lowering agents; the strongest such evidence currently exists for ezetimibe added to statins.[52]

Extreme hypertriglyceridemia (>1,000 mg/dL) predisposes to pancreatitis more than ASCVD; hence, in patients with such severe elevations, the need for aggressive triglyceride lowering with fibrate drugs in addition to nutritional modification and optimization of hyperglycemia to prevent an acute pancreatitis attack supersedes any ASCVD concerns. Lesser degrees of hypertriglyceridemia (150–500 mg/dL) are much more common in diabetes and confer increased ASCVD risk (in close association with other ASCVD risk factors such as low HDL cholesterol, pro-atherogenic LDL particles, and many other features of insulin resistance and the metabolic syndrome).[53] ATP-III advocates the use of non–HDL cholesterol (total cholesterol minus HDL cholesterol) as a secondary target of lipid-lowering therapy for patients with triglyceride levels >200 mg/dL after the LDL cholesterol target has been achieved.[46] The goal for non–HDL cholesterol is <30 mg/dL above the patient's LDL cholesterol target for the risk category, and lowering of non–HDL cholesterol should begin with further intensification of the patient's statin therapy. Although fibrates are known to be cardioprotective,[54,55] their evidence basis for ASCVD risk reduction is weaker than that of statins,[56] so intensification of statins is still the preferred strategy to achieve the non–HDL cholesterol goal. If statin monotherapy is insufficient to achieve both LDL and non–HDL cholesterol targets, combination therapy with addition of ezetimibe or fibrates may be considered, particularly fibrates for male patients with elevated triglycerides and reduced HDL cholesterol levels.[49] It should be noted that adding a fibrate to a statin substantially increases liver and muscle toxicity risk and thus requires closer monitoring[57]; that fenofibrate is preferred over gemfibrozil because of its more favorable interaction profile with statins[58]; and that, as yet, there is no clear evidence of additive ASCVD risk reduction when fibrates are added to statins.[59]

NEPHROPATHY

Markers of diabetic nephropathy include declining renal function, as determined by a calculation of estimated glomerular filtration rate (eGFR), and increased albuminuria, as determined by a ratio of urine albumin to urine creatinine concentrations (UACR); both markers should be assessed regularly, since both can reflect progression of nephropathy independently of each other. The ADA had previously distinguished microalbuminuria, defined as a UACR of 30–300 mg/g of urine creatinine, from macroalbuminuria or clinical albuminuria, defined as a UACR >300 mg/g of urine creatinine. However, current guidelines only recognize the entire continuum of any degree of albuminuria (defined as any UACR ≥30 mg/g), since they represent the same underlying disease process.[60]

Many studies have evaluated the effects of either ACE inhibitors or angiotensin receptor blockers (ARBs) on renal disease in diabetic patients. Studies on patients with macroalbuminuria, many of whom also had renal insufficiency, used a primary end point of a doubling of serum creatinine levels and secondary end points of dialysis, renal transplant, or death. In randomized control trials of both ACE inhibitors[61] and ARBs,[62,63] these end points were significantly reduced compared to placebo. The effects were not attributable to BP lowering because either BP levels were kept the same in both the intervention and control groups[61] or the benefits were independent of BP changes.[62,63] Many smaller studies also support these conclusions,[64] and more recent meta-analyses also confirm the superiority of ACE inhibitors or ARBs for preservation of renal function compared to other classes of agents.[65,66] However, the combined use of ACE inhibitors and ARBs together do not provide any additive protection, and may be associated with adverse events (hyperkalemia and/or acute kidney injury).[67]

ACE inhibitors and ARBs also reduced the progression of microalbuminuria to macroalbuminuria and increased the return of microalbuminuria to normoalbuminuria.[64] These effects were independent of changes in BP. Studies in normotensive type 1[68] and type 2[69] diabetic patients, in which an ACE inhibitor significantly decreased the development of macroalbuminuria from microalbuminuria, prove this point. When the ACE inhibitor was discontinued (by patient choice), microalbuminuria returned,[70] showing that the improvement was not due to natural variability. Finally, a meta-regression analysis showed that although lowering BP decreased proteinuria and increased glomerular filtration rate, ACE inhibitors had an additional beneficial effect independent of their effect on BP.[71] A systematic review has also confirmed the superiority of ACE inhibitors and ARBs over other agents as well as placebo on reducing progression to macroalbuminuria.[65]

Based on these data, the ADA[60] recommends annual assessments of UACR and eGFR (for patients with type 1 diabetes, starting ≥5 years after initial diabetes diagnosis), and unless contraindicated, patients with confirmed albuminuria (based on 2 out of 3 determinations performed within a 3- to 6-month period, because mild albuminuria can be transient) should be given either an ACE inhibitor or ARB, regardless of their BP. Furthermore, unless contraindicated, for diabetic individuals with hypertension, one of these agents should be part of the patient's anti-hypertension treatment regimen. However, there is no evidence that ACE inhibitors or ARBs are preventive in normotensive diabetic patients without albuminuria, so routine use in such cases is not recommended.[72]

HYPERTENSION

The patterns of hypertension between type 1 and type 2 diabetic patients are different. In the former, hypertension usually only occurs after patients develop renal disease. In the latter, hypertension is up to three times more common than in age- and sex-matched nondiabetic individuals and is strongly associated with insulin resistance, so it is frequently present when type 2 diabetes is diagnosed. Evidence supports the benefits of intensive BP control for diabetic patients. In the Systolic Hypertension in the Elderly Program (SHEP), intensively treated diabetic patients achieved systolic and diastolic BP levels of 9.8 and 2.2 mmHg, respectively, below those of the usual care group, and had a 34% lower rate of cardiovascular events, a 20% lower rate of strokes, and a 26% lower total mortality rate.[73] In the Systolic Hypertension in Europe (Syst-Eur) study,[74] actively treated diabetic subjects achieved systolic and diastolic BP levels of 8.6 and 3.9 mmHg, respectively, below the levels of placebo-treated subjects, and had a 70% lower cardiovascular mortality rate, a 65% lower cardiovascular event rate, a 73% lower rate of stroke, and a 55% lower total mortality rate. In the UKPDS, intensively treated subjects achieved a mean BP of 144/82 mmHg, compared to 154/87 mmHg in the less intensively treated group, and had a 34% lower rate of cardiovascular events and a 44% lower rate of stroke.[75]

Additional studies assessed specific BP targets. In the Hypertension Optimal Treatment (HOT) study, patients were randomly assigned to target diastolic BP levels of 90, 85, or 80 mmHg.[76] Among the full study cohort, the group targeting 80 mmHg (achieving a mean of 81 mmHg) had a 51% lower rate of cardiovascular events and a 44% lower rate of cardiovascular deaths compared to the group targeting 90 mmHg (achieving a mean of 85 mmHg). However, the analysis of the diabetic subgroup in this study was post hoc and represented only 8% of the entire study cohort. In the Appropriate Blood Pressure Control in Diabetes (ABCD) trial,[77] the intensive treatment group targeting a diastolic BP of 75 mmHg (and achieving a mean BP of 132/78 mmHg), compared to the moderate control group targeting a diastolic BP of 80–89 mmHg (and achieving a mean BP of 138/86 mmHg), had a 49% lower total mortality rate, but there was no difference in cardiovascular mortality to explain it.

Until recently, the ADA and the National Kidney Foundation had recommended a more stringent BP target of <130/80 mmHg for diabetic patients, based on the prospective epidemiological association between cardiovascular mortality and BP as low as 115/75 mmHg,[78] and the additive risk conferred by hypertension coexisting with diabetes. However, more recent interventional studies did not support the use of such an intensive target. In the large ACCORD-BP trial, intensive treatment targeting a systolic BP <120 mmHg (achieving a mean of 119 mmHg), compared to moderate treatment targeting systolic BP <140 mmHg (achieving a mean of 133 mmHg), failed to significantly reduce a composite measure of cardio-vascular events or total mortality; only strokes were reduced by 41%, but serious adverse events also increased by 30%.[79] In the ADVANCE-BP trial, treatment that achieved a mean BP of 135/74 mmHg, as compared to the placebo group that achieved 140/75 mmHg, resulted in a significant 18% reduction of cardiovascular deaths and a 14% reduction in total mortality, but only a nonsignificant 8% reduc-tion in a composite measure of major macrovascular events.[80] After 6 more years of follow-up, when mean BPs no longer differed between groups, the cardiovas-cular and total mortality rates had been attenuated (down to 12% and 9%, respec-tively), albeit they were still statistically significant.[81] Accordingly, a recent meta-analysis of the available evidence to date found no significant overall reduc-tion of MIs or mortality with intensive BP targets and found only a 1% reduction in the absolute risk of stroke.[82] Meta-analysis evidence does, however, still support the benefits of a 140/90 mmHg target for diabetic patients.[83] Therefore, consis-tent with the Eighth Joint National Committee (JNC8) recommendations for the general population,[84] the ADA currently recommends targeting systolic BP <140 mmHg and diastolic BP <90 mmHg for all patients with diabetes.[49] However, the ADA also recognizes the option of the more intensive target of <130/80 mmHg for individuals at high risk of cardiovascular disease if it can be achieved without undue burden.[49]

Intensive BP reductions should be maintained if the cardiovascular benefits are to be sustained. This result is seen in long-term follow-up studies such as those in the ADVANCE-BP trial,[81] which found attenuation of cardiovascular benefit as the BP difference waned over time, or the UKPDS, which found almost complete loss of cardiovascular benefit by about 10 years after the BP treatment difference was lost.[85] It should also be emphasized that more intensive BP control may also have greater benefits on the microvascular complications of diabetes, particularly in patients with renal insufficiency for whom BP control is the most important factor in preserving renal function.[86] In the ABCD trial, moderate BP control among hypertensive patients slowed the progression of microvascular outcomes, at least as well as intensive BP control, but the trial included only 470 subjects.[77] In the larger UKPDS (1,148 subjects), a composite measure of retinopathy pro-gression and renal failure was reduced by 37% with intensive control compared to less intensive control.[75] Also, in ACCORD-BP (4,733 subjects), albuminuria was reduced with intensive BP control compared to moderate control, although declines in GFR were not slowed.[79]

RETINOPATHY

There are two main reasons for screening for diabetic retinopathy: first, the pro-cess before visual loss is usually asymptomatic and, second, laser photocoagula-tion surgery effectively stabilizes vision (but does not restore it), while anti-vascular endothelial growth factor (anti-VEGF) agents may reverse it.[60] Two large randomized trials firmly established the beneficial effects of laser photoco-agulation surgery for severe diabetic retinopathy (but not for mild or moderate disease). In the Diabetic Retinopathy Study,[87] pan-retinal photocoagulation decreased the incidence of severe visual loss (i.e., best acuity of 5/200 or worse) by 50% during a 6-year follow-up, starting almost immediately. The results of focal photocoagulation for macular edema (the most common retinal cause for visual loss in type 2 diabetic patients) in the Early Treatment Diabetic Retinopathy Study (ETDRS)[88] were similar. The end point was a 50% deterioration in vision evaluated by an acuity chart (e.g., 20/40 to 20/80). After 3 years, 12% of the treated eyes compared with 24% of the untreated eyes had deteriorated to that extent. Further analysis revealed that only eyes with "clinically significant macular edema" needed to be treated because the rate of visual loss was very low in eyes with milder macular changes, and there was no evidence of benefit from treatment of this earlier process. Retinal thickening that occurs at or near the center of the macula is the hallmark of clinically significant macular edema. Unfortunately, this condition can only be assessed by stereo contact lens biomicroscopy and stereo photography, procedures not available to non-ophthalmologists (although exudates in the macular area almost always predict retinal thickening). To complicate matters further, initial visual acuity does not help select patients for further investigation. Even patients with normal visual acuity, but with clinically significant macular edema, were helped by focal macular photocoagulation.

Thus, the ADA recommends that yearly eye examinations be performed, starting at the time of diagnosis (within 5 years of diagnosis for type 1 diabetic patients)[60] to detect macular edema that would benefit from laser photocoagulation surgery, with or without adjunctive treatment using intra-vitreal anti-vascular endothelial growth factor (anti-VEGF) agents.[89] Patients with normal annual retina examinations may be subsequently followed at intervals of every 2–3 years.[90] Although the ADA emphasizes that comprehensive eye examinations should be performed by eye care professionals, we[91] (and others[92]) have previously shown that screening with funduscopic photographs taken with a non-mydriatic retina camera, with images interpreted by providers who are familiar with diabetic retinopathy, was highly sensitive and cost-effective for the detection of any serious diabetic retinopathy that would warrant an ophthalmology referral. Although the ADA still recommends surveillance with comprehensive eye exams, for resource-limited health care settings where appropriate eye care professionals may not be as readily available, funduscopic photography represents an alternative yet effective screening strategy for diabetic retinopathy that is supported by the ADA.[60]

PERIPHERAL NEUROPATHY AND FOOT EXAMINATION

Diabetic peripheral neuropathy (DPN) in the lower extremities can present heterogeneously, either as tingling and pain (dysesthesia) and/or numbness (hypoesthesia), progressing to loss of sensation (anesthesia). Thus, in addition to soliciting symptoms of lower-extremity pain that may warrant analgesic treatment, the ADA recommends that testing for the sensory loss of DPN using an objective method such as the 5.07 Semmes-Weinstein nylon monofilament[93] should be performed at least annually.[60] Loss of sensation to the 10 g of pressure of the monofilament, when it is applied to at least four weight-bearing points on the plantar surface of each foot (e.g., toes, metatarsal heads), has been shown to prospectively predict the progression to foot ulceration.[94,95] If such early sensory loss can be identified through regular testing, intensive glycemic control can also be instituted early. Tight glycemic control has been shown to prevent and delay progression of DPN in type 1 diabetes[20] and (albeit less convincingly) in type 2 diabetes.[21,23]

Despite some encouraging recent trends, rates of nontraumatic lower-extremity amputations in diabetic individuals remain 8–10 times higher than in comparable nondiabetic individuals,[9,96] and 85% of lower-extremity amputations in diabetic patients are secondary to foot ulcers.[93] Early signs of foot pathology, such as areas of erythema, warmth, and/or calluses, reflect the effects of increased pressure predisposing to eventual ulceration; regular foot examinations should be performed to detect these early signs before ulceration occurs. Proper patient education regarding regular foot monitoring, foot care, and proper footwear is also important,[93] particularly for patients with high-risk feet (e.g., prior ulcers or amputations, insensate feet, coexisting deformities, or peripheral arterial disease).

ASPIRIN

Randomized controlled trials of aspirin for primary prevention of ASCVD, specifically in diabetic patients, have generally failed to convincingly demonstrate significant reductions in ASCVD outcomes.[97–99] However, a large meta-analysis of antiplatelet therapies for the secondary prevention of serious vascular events (defined as MIs, strokes, or vascular deaths) found a significant 22–25% relative risk reduction with the use of aspirin,[100] using doses between 75 and 162 mg daily that were at least as effective as higher doses. There was also a 60% increase in the relative risk of extra-cranial bleeding and a 22% increase in the relative risk of hemorrhagic strokes, but in terms of absolute event rates, the reductions in occlusive events far outweighed the increases in bleeding and hemorrhagic strokes (10–13% vs. 0.7–1.1%, respectively).

A subsequent meta-analysis that included both primary and secondary prevention studies of aspirin on serious vascular events[101] found a 12% relative risk reduction with aspirin use among the primary prevention studies (mostly due to a ~20% relative risk reduction of nonfatal MIs), but also a 54% increase in the relative risk of gastrointestinal and extra-cranial bleeding (although the absolute reduction of occlusive events again far outweighed the absolute increases in bleeding episodes). Among these primary prevention studies, there was no difference in the relative risk reduction for the subgroup with diabetes compared to nondiabetic individuals. Among the secondary prevention studies in this meta-analysis, a 22% relative risk reduction similar to that of the previous meta-analysis was seen, but bleeding events were inconsistently reported among these studies.

Thus, the benefits of aspirin for ASCVD prevention must be weighed against an increased bleeding risk, with the risk-benefit balance being more favorable for secondary prevention than that for primary prevention. The most recent standards of care from the ADA[49] state that, unless contraindicated, low-dose (75–162 mg/day) aspirin should be used for secondary ASCVD prevention in all diabetic patients with a history of ASCVD. Its use is also reasonable for diabetic adults with no previous ASCVD history (i.e., primary prevention) who are at increased ASCVD risk (which includes most diabetic individuals age ≥50 years who have one or more of the following major risk factors: smoking, hypertension, dyslipidemia, family history of premature ASCVD, or albuminuria) and who are not at increased risk for bleeding. Aspirin is currently not recommended for diabetic individuals at low ASCVD risk (defined as individuals age <50 years with no other major ASCVD risk factors), since the potential adverse effects from bleeding offset the potential benefits. Clinical judgment should be used for individuals who do not meet either of these criteria (e.g., younger patients with risk factors or older patients without risk factors).

Aspirin use does not increase the risk of retinal or vitreous hemorrhage.[97] Contraindications to aspirin use include aspirin allergy, a known bleeding tendency, anticoagulant therapy, recent gastrointestinal bleeding, history of a hemorrhagic stroke, and clinically active hepatitis. Use of enteric-coated aspirin formulations do not reduce the risk of gastrointestinal bleeding.[102] Clopidogrel is an alternative antiplatelet agent for aspirin-intolerant individuals that may be at least as effective as aspirin for ASCVD risk reduction in diabetic patients[103] as well as in the overall population.[104]

SMOKING CESSATION

Despite the large body of evidence irrefutably establishing the causal relationship between smoking and health risks, and role of smoking as the leading cause of preventable diseases and deaths in the U.S., approximately 18% of the U.S adult population, or 42.1 million people, still smoke cigarettes.[105] The prevalence of smoking among patients with diabetes is believed to mirror that of the general population.[106] According to one national survey, among all smokers in 2010, over two-thirds report wanting to quit, and 44% attempted to quit within the past year, but only 4–7% are successful each year.[107] Despite this, among current smokers attending outpatient physician visits, only 20.9% received tobacco counseling from their physician, and only 7.6% received a prescription or order for a medication associated with tobacco cessation.[107] For diabetic patients who smoke, not only are cardiovascular risks compounded, but smoking also worsens insulin resistance[108] and glycemic control[109] and increases the development of microvascular complications.[110,111] Conversely, smoking cessation may be associated with improved glycemic control[112,113] and amelioration of some microvascular complications.[113] And contrary to popular belief, after smoking cessation, weight gain is not inevitable,[114] can be minimized using appropriate strategies,[114,115] and, if weight gain does occur, it does not attenuate the reduction of cardiovascular risk associated with smoking cessation.[116] Thus, smoking cessation is critically important and must be emphasized and encouraged for all diabetic patients who smoke. Use of electronic cigarettes (e-cigarettes) should also be discouraged, as there are no data supporting their role as a more favorable alternative to cigarettes, nor as an aid for cigarette smoking cessation.[117] Patient support through counseling with or without pharmacological aids should be provided when needed.

Based on the foregoing data, the ADA has recommended guidelines for diabetes care that, if met, would markedly reduce the complications of diabetes (Table 1.1). When considering guidelines, it is important to distinguish between process

Table 1.1. Recommended ADA Treatment Guidelines

Guideline	Frequency	Goal
1. A1C	*At least twice each year* if goal attained *Quarterly* if goal not attained or if adjusting treatment	<7.0% (Lower or higher goal may be reasonable for select patients)
2. BP	Every routine visit	Systolic <140 mmHg Diastolic <90 mmHg (a lower goal of <130/80 mmHg may be reasonable for select patients)
3. Dyslipidemia	Lipid profile at diabetes diagnosis, initial evaluation, and every 5 years thereafter, or more frequently if indicated* (for patients not taking a statin)	Use of a statin (with or without ezetimibe; see Chapter 4) with LDL cholesterol–lowering intensity appropriate to the patient's risk profile
4. Aspirin (75–162 mg)	Prescribe if age ≥50 years and at least one major ASCVD risk factor; no contraindications	Maintain
5. Nephropathy	*At least once each year*: UACR and estimated glomerular filtration rate (eGFR), starting at diagnosis in all type 2 diabetic patients (starting 5 years after diabetes diagnosis for type 1 diabetic patients), and all patients with concurrent hypertension	In patients with hypertension, use of an ACE inhibitor or ARB if albuminuria is present Optimize BP Optimize glucose
6. Retinopathy	Comprehensive dilated eye exam (or fundus photograph with proper image interpretation if dilated eye exam is otherwise unobtainable) at diagnosis in all type 2 diabetic patients (starting within 5 years after diabetes diagnosis for type 1 diabetic patients)† *At least annually* thereafter May reduce to every 2 years if normal	Optimize BP Optimize glucose Ophthalmology referral for laser photocoagulation therapy and/or other intra-vitreal anti-VEGF therapies
7. Peripheral neuropathy	Sensory testing (e.g., Semmes-Weinstein 5.07 [10-g] monofilament) plus at least one of the following: pinprick, temperature, or vibration testing; at diabetes diagnosis in all type 2 diabetic patients (starting 5 years after diabetes diagnosis for type 1 diabetic patients) *At least annually* thereafter	Optimize glucose Control neuropathic pain if present
8. Foot care	*At least annual* comprehensive foot exam (including vascular status), but feet should be inspected at *every visit*, particularly if ulcers, amputations, peripheral arterial disease, or deformities are present, or if insensate feet are present; refer to foot care specialists as appropriate	Provide general preventive foot care education; specialized therapeutic footwear recommended for high-risk patients Prevent ulceration or foot deformities
9. Smoking cessation/ prevention	*Routinely* counsel	Avoidance/cessation

*As recommended by ADA,[49] although we prefer to routinely monitor the lipid profile more frequently, e.g., at least every 1–2 years.
†The presence of glaucoma or cataracts would further justify eye exams by a qualified eye care professional.

measures and outcome measures. Process measures are the number of tests or examinations carried out per period of time or whether an indicated treatment is given. Outcome measures are the actual results of the test or the effect of the treatment. Unfortunately, simply meeting process measure goals may or may not translate into improvement of outcome measures[118,119] (e.g., frequent measurements of A1C levels do not necessarily lead to lowered glycemia).

RATIONALE FOR USING TREATMENT ALGORITHMS

Despite some modest improvements over the past few decades, many diabetic patients still do not meet the recommended goals outlined in Table 1.1. According to statistics from the U.S. National Health and Nutrition Examination Survey (NHANES), the ADA glycemic goal of A1C <7.0%, met by only 43% in 1994, had increased to only 52% by 2010, meaning that roughly half of diabetic patients still remain suboptimally controlled.[120] The LDL cholesterol goal of <100 mg/dL was met by only 10% in 1994 and dramatically increased to 56% by 2010. However, this result still indicates that roughly half of diabetic patients remain suboptimally controlled for their dyslipidemia (according to previously recommended LDL cholesterol targets). These data parallel the dramatic rise in the use of statins (from 4% in 1994 up to 51% in 2010), which by current guidelines should now be a standard treatment for the vast majority of diabetic patients. And using the currently recommended BP goal of <140/90 mmHg, 62% met the target in 1994, while 72% met the target in 2010, again improving over time, but still leaving over one-quarter of all diabetic individuals suboptimally controlled by current BP recommendations (as expected, when using the prior BP goal of <130/80 mmHg, only 51% met this target in 2010). However, particularly alarming is the fact that the percentage of diabetic patients meeting all three goals simultaneously (A1C <7.0%, LDL cholesterol <100 mg/dL, and BP <130/80 mmHg), as would be expected with ideal management, was a dismal 1.7% in 1994, but had only increased to 19% by 2010.[120]

In an NHANES analysis of ACE inhibitor or ARB use among diabetic patients age ≥55 years, in which 41% had albuminuria and 83% had hypertension as an indication for an ACE inhibitor or ARB (and upon adding ASCVD, 100% had at least one indication), only 43% of individuals overall were actually taking an ACE inhibitor or ARB.[121] Among the highest-risk individuals with four or more indications, the rate was still only 53%. Hypertension as an indication was associated with greater usage compared to no hypertension (48% vs. 21%), but albuminuria as an indication was not significantly associated with greater usage compared to no albuminuria (47% vs. 43%).[121] As for smoking cessation, pooled data from the Behavioral Risk Factor Surveillance System (BRFSS) spanning 2001–2010 showed that mean rates of smoking cessation in diabetic individuals actually lagged slightly behind that of nondiabetic individuals (0.25 vs. 0.67% per year, respectively).[122] And despite the additive risk of smoking and diabetes, the trends of smoking and smoking cessation over 10 years were largely no different between diabetic and nondiabetic individuals.[122]

Other process measures related to current diabetes management recommendations also leave much room for improvement. Data combined from the 2005, 2007, and 2009 BRFSS showed that only 62.5% of age-appropriate U.S. adults with diabetes (i.e., individuals who would benefit) used aspirin daily or near daily.[123] Additional data from the 2009–2010 BRFSS show that only 63% of U.S. adult diabetic patients received an annual eye exam, only 67.5% had at least one annual foot exam, only 68.5% had an A1C determination at least twice in the past year, only 57% had ever attended a diabetes self-management class, and only 50% received an annual flu vaccine.[124] Thus, at least one-third of all U.S. diabetic patients are still failing to meet one or more ADA management recommendations.

An important barrier to good diabetes care is the lack of timely and appropriate treatment decisions. This occurrence may be due in part to the lack of time that physicians have to spend with patients and not necessarily related to clinical inertia (as defined below). A primary care physician typically has 10–15 min with each patient, and in that time, attention needs to be paid to all of the process measures listed in Table 1.1. These issues often may not receive the attention they deserve because most are not typically associated with symptoms, so the patient's other symptomatic complaints that are unrelated to diabetes often take priority. Studies in actual practice settings have shown that higher patient volume[125] and more patient concerns[126] can interfere with appropriate intensification of glucose-lowering therapy. Moreover, patients are often seen at intervals of approximately every 3 months, which permits glycemia, lipids, and BP to remain out of control for longer time periods between physician encounters.

However, clinical inertia—the lack of an appropriate treatment decision when the patient's clinical situation indicates that one should be made—is often another major factor. For example, diabetic patients treated with a single oral agent in a large U.S. HMO had a mean of 4.5 A1C determinations >8.0%, and a final spike to >9.0%, before a second oral agent was added on average 30 months later.[127] When followed prospectively through the typical progression from nonpharmacologic therapy to monotherapy to combination therapy, these patients spent nearly 5 years with A1C levels >8.0% and ~10 years with values >7.0% before starting insulin.[128] The transition from oral agents to insulin therapy is particularly prone to clinical inertia. In a longitudinal follow-up study, less than half of patients failing to maintain control on combination oral agents (A1C >8.0%) transitioned to insulin over a period of 4.5 years.[129] Clinical inertia is not limited to the U.S., but also affects diabetes care in other developed nations. In the U.K., there are similar delays in starting insulin,[130] and a large survey recently found that among those with A1C >8.0%, median time to the addition of a second agent, a third agent, or insulin was 1.6, 6.9, and 6.0 years, respectively.[131] In Canada, even under a specialist's care, less than half of patients with A1C >8.0% had their treatment intensified.[132] Another recent national survey found only 53% of diabetic patients in Canada achieved an A1C <7.0%, only 64% achieved an LDL cholesterol <100 mg/dL, only 74% were receiving statins (which were not used in 43% of patients with LDL cholesterol above target), 46% had a BP that was above target, and only 21% achieved all three targets (A1C, BP, and LDL cholesterol) simultaneously.[133] Even within U.S. academic medical centers,[134] A1C, BP <130/80 mmHg, and LDL cholesterol goals were met by only 34, 33, and 46%, respectively; only 10% met all three goals simultaneously. Only 40% with A1C above goal had their treatment intensified, and only 10% and 5.6% of untreated patients above BP and LDL cholesterol goals, respectively, had treatment initiated.[134]

The factors that underlie clinical inertia are complex but involve physician factors (e.g., knowledge, acceptability, or applicability of guidelines; uncertainty regarding individualized decisions or biological outcomes), patient factors (e.g., preferences/beliefs, treatment adherence, health literacy, self-efficacy, and empowerment), and/or system factors (e.g., competing demands, health care system, and organizational constraints).[135] To the extent that our treatment algorithms for glycemia, lipids, and BP as described in Chapters 3, 4, and 5 will help to overcome some of the physician factors (and possibly some system factors, if they can be incorporated and automated within electronic health record systems to facilitate decision-making through physician reminders, alerts, and/or feedback), they will help to ensure that timely and appropriate clinical decisions are made, leading to improved diabetes outcomes, particularly within time- or resource-constrained health care settings.

For the past 33 years, the first author has trained and supervised nurses, nurse practitioners, pharmacists, and physician assistants to use these algorithms in caring for people with diabetes, with gratifying results. For instance, in an especially challenging, medically underserved minority population, a dedicated registered nurse following these algorithms in 545 patients for 9–12 months achieved a mean A1C level of 7.1%, with 57% meeting the ADA A1C goal of <7.0%, 87% meeting the LDL cholesterol goal of <100 mg/dL, 90% meeting the systolic BP goal of <130 mmHg, and 95% meeting the diastolic BP goal of <80 mmHg.[136] A subsequent application of the same algorithms for 9–12 months in a similar population used an integrated model wherein the registered nurse provider was placed within the family medicine clinic and was supervised by the primary care physicians at the site. The physicians referred their patients to her care. In this setting, a substantially higher baseline A1C of 11.1% was successfully lowered to a comparable 7.2%, 49% met the ADA A1C goal (up from a baseline rate of 0%), 96% met the LDL cholesterol goal, and 90 and 95% met the systolic and diastolic BP goals, respectively.[137]

Thus, if providers follow the treatment algorithms described in Chapters 3, 4, and 5, clinical inertia may be eliminated, timely and appropriate treatment decisions will be made, and patients will escape or at least markedly attenuate the potentially devastating complications of diabetes.

REFERENCES

1. American Diabetes Association. Economic costs of diabetes in the U.S. in 2012. *Diabetes Care* 2013;36:1033–1046

2. Zhang X, Saaddine JB, Chou CF, et al. Prevalence of diabetic retinopathy in the United States, 2005–2008. *JAMA* 2010;304:649–656

3. Saran R, Li Y, Robinson B, et al. U.S. Renal Data System 2014 Annual Data Report: Epidemiology of kidney disease in the United States. *Am J Kidney Dis* 2015;66 (Suppl. 1):S1–S305

4. Pecoraro RE, Reiber GE, Burgess EM. Pathways to diabetic limb amputation: basis for prevention. *Diabetes Care* 1990;13:513–521

5. Global Lower Extremity Amputation Study Group. Epidemiology of lower extremity amputation in centres in Europe, North America and East Asia. *Br J Surg* 2000;87:328–337

6. Kannel WB, McGee DL. Diabetes and cardiovascular risk factors: the Framingham study. *Circulation* 1979;59:8–13

7. Hewitt J, Castilla Guerra L, Fernandez-Moreno M del C, Sierra C. Diabetes and stroke prevention: a review. *Stroke Res Treat* 2012:673187

8. Marso SP, Hiatt WR. Peripheral arterial disease in patients with diabetes. *J Am Coll Cardiol* 2006;47:921–929

9. Gregg EW, Li Y, Wang J, et al. Changes in diabetes-related complications in the United States, 1990–2010. *N Engl J Med* 2014;370:1514–1523

10. Skyler JS. Diabetic complications: the importance of glucose control. *Endocrinol Metab Clin North Am* 1996;25:243–254

11. Krolewski AS, Laffel LM, Krolewski M, Quinn M, Warram JH. Glycosylated hemoglobin and the risk of microalbuminuria in patients with insulin-dependent diabetes mellitus. *N Engl J Med* 1995;332:1251–1255

12. Warram JH, Scott LJ, Hanna LS, et al. Progression of microalbuminuria to proteinuria in type 1 diabetes: nonlinear relationship with hyperglycemia. *Diabetes* 2000;49:94–100

13. Ohkubo Y, Kishikawa H, Araki E, et al. Intensive insulin therapy prevents the progression of diabetic microvascular complications in Japanese patients with non-insulin-dependent diabetes mellitus: a randomized prospective 6-year study. *Diabetes Res Clin Pract* 1995;28:103–117

14. Tanaka Y, Atsumi Y, Matsuoka K, et al. Role of glycemic control and blood pressure in the development and progression of nephropathy in elderly Japanese NIDDM patients. *Diabetes Care* 1998;21:116–120

15. Diabetes Control and Complications Trial Research Group. The effect of intensive treatment of diabetes on the development and progression of long-term complications in insulin-dependent diabetes mellitus. *N Engl J Med* 1993;329:977–986

16. Diabetes Control and Complications Trial/Epidemiology of Diabetes Interventions and Complications Research Group. Retinopathy and nephropathy in patients with type 1 diabetes four years after a trial of intensive therapy. *N Engl J Med* 2000;342:381–389

17. Martin CL, Albers J, Herman WH, et al. Neuropathy among the diabetes control and complications trial cohort 8 years after trial completion. *Diabetes Care* 2006;29:340–344

18. Diabetes Control and Complications Trial (DCCT)/Epidemiology of Diabetes Interventions and Complications (EDIC) Research Group. Effect of

intensive diabetes therapy on the progression of diabetic retinopathy in patients with type 1 diabetes: 18 years of follow-up in the DCCT/EDIC. *Diabetes* 2015;64:631–642

19. DCCT/EDIC Research Group. Effect of intensive diabetes treatment on albuminuria in type 1 diabetes: long-term follow-up of the Diabetes Control and Complications Trial and Epidemiology of Diabetes Interventions and Complications study. *Lancet Diabetes Endocrinol* 2014;2:793–800

20. Martin CL, Albers JW, Pop-Busui R. Neuropathy and related findings in the Diabetes Control and Complications Trial/Epidemiology of Diabetes Interventions and Complications Study. *Diabetes Care* 2014;37:31–38

21. UK Prospective Diabetes Study (UKPDS) Group. Intensive blood-glucose control with sulphonylureas or insulin compared with conventional treatment and risk of complications in patients with type 2 diabetes (UKPDS 33). *Lancet* 1998;352:837–853

22. Holman RR, Paul SK, Bethel MA, et al. 10-year follow-up of intensive glucose control in type 2 diabetes. *N Engl J Med* 2008;359:1577–1589

23. Ismail-Beigi F, Craven T, Banerji MA, et al. Effect of intensive treatment of hyperglycaemia on microvascular outcomes in type 2 diabetes: an analysis of the ACCORD randomised trial. *Lancet* 2010;376:419–430

24. Action to Control Cardiovascular Risk in Diabetes Follow-On (ACCORDION) Eye Study Group, The Action to Control Cardiovascular Risk in Diabetes Follow-On (ACCORDION) Study Group. Persistent effects of intensive glycemic control on retinopathy in type 2 diabetes in the Action to Control Cardiovascular Risk in Diabetes (ACCORD) Follow-On Study. *Diabetes Care* 2016;39:1089–1100

25. Patel A, MacMahon S, Chalmers J, et al. Intensive blood glucose control and vascular outcomes in patients with type 2 diabetes. *N Engl J Med* 2008;358:2560–2572

26. Duckworth W, Abraira C, Moritz T, et al. Glucose control and vascular complications in veterans with type 2 diabetes. *N Engl J Med* 2009;360:129–139

27. Gerstein HC, Miller ME, Byington RP, et al. Effects of intensive glucose lowering in type 2 diabetes. *N Engl J Med* 2008;358:2545–2559

28. Khaw KT, Wareham N, Luben R, et al. Glycated haemoglobin, diabetes, and mortality in men in Norfolk cohort of the European Prospective Investigation of Cancer and Nutrition (EPIC-Norfolk). *BMJ* 2001;322:15–18

29. Selvin E, Coresh J, Golden SH, et al. Glycemic control and coronary heart disease risk in persons with and without diabetes: the Atherosclerosis Risk in Communities Study. *Arch Intern Med* 2005;165:1910–1916

30. Stettler C, Allemann S, Juni P, et al. Glycemic control and macrovascular disease in types 1 and 2 diabetes mellitus: meta-analysis of randomized trials. *Am Heart J* 2006;152:27–38

31. Nathan DM, Cleary PA, Backlund JY, et al. Intensive diabetes treatment and cardiovascular disease in patients with type 1 diabetes. *N Engl J Med* 2005;353:2643–2653

32. Nathan DM, Zinman B, Cleary PA, et al. Modern-day clinical course of type 1 diabetes mellitus after 30 years' duration: the Diabetes Control and Complications Trial/Epidemiology of Diabetes Interventions and Complications and Pittsburgh Epidemiology of Diabetes Complications experience (1983–2005). *Arch Intern Med* 2009;169:1307–1316

33. Diabetes Control and Complications Trial (DCCT)/Epidemiology of Diabetes Interventions and Complications (EDIC) Study Research Group. Intensive diabetes treatment and cardiovascular outcomes in type 1 diabetes: the DCCT/EDIC Study 30-year follow-up. *Diabetes Care* 2016;39:686–693

34. Writing Group for the DCCT/EDIC Research Group. Association between 7 years of intensive treatment of type 1 diabetes and long-term mortality. *JAMA* 2015;313:45–53

35. ACCORD Study Group. Long-term effects of intensive glucose lowering on cardiovascular outcomes. *N Engl J Med* 2011;364:818–828

36. ACCORD Study Group. Nine-year effects of 3.7 years of intensive glycemic control on cardiovascular outcomes. *Diabetes Care* 2016;39:701–708

37. Skyler JS, Bergenstal R, Bonow RO, et al. Intensive glycemic control and the prevention of cardiovascular events: implications of the ACCORD, ADVANCE, and VA diabetes trials: a position statement of the American Diabetes Association and a scientific statement of the American College of Cardiology Foundation and the American Heart Association. *Diabetes Care* 2009;32:187–192

38. Turnbull FM, Abraira C, Anderson RJ, et al. Intensive glucose control and macrovascular outcomes in type 2 diabetes. *Diabetologia* 2009;52:2288–2298

39. American Diabetes Association. Glycemic targets. *Diabetes Care* 2016;39(Suppl. 1):S39–S46

40. Baigent C, Keech A, Kearney PM, et al. Efficacy and safety of cholesterol-lowering treatment: prospective meta-analysis of data from 90,056 participants in 14 randomised trials of statins. *Lancet* 2005;366:1267–1278

41. Baigent C, Blackwell L, Emberson J, et al. Efficacy and safety of more intensive lowering of LDL cholesterol: a meta-analysis of data from 170,000 participants in 26 randomised trials. *Lancet* 2010;376:1670–1681

42. Kearney PM, Blackwell L, Collins R, et al. Efficacy of cholesterol-lowering therapy in 18,686 people with diabetes in 14 randomised trials of statins: a meta-analysis. *Lancet* 2008;371:117–125

43. Costa J, Borges M, David C, Vaz Carneiro A. Efficacy of lipid lowering drug treatment for diabetic and non-diabetic patients: meta-analysis of randomised controlled trials. *BMJ* 2006;332:1115–1124

44. Brandle M, Davidson MB, Schriger DL, Lorber B, Herman WH. Cost effectiveness of statin therapy for the primary prevention of major coronary events in individuals with type 2 diabetes. *Diabetes Care* 2003;26:1796–1801

45. American Diabetes Association. Standards of medical care in diabetes, 2014. *Diabetes Care* 2014;37(Suppl. 1):S14–S80

46. Expert Panel on Detection, Evaluation, and Treatment of High Blood Cholesterol in Adults. Executive summary of the Third Report of the National Cholesterol Education Program (NCEP) Expert Panel on Detection, Evaluation, and Treatment of High Blood Cholesterol in Adults (Adult Treatment Panel III). *JAMA* 2001;285:2486–2497

47. Grundy SM, Cleeman JI, Merz CN, et al. Implications of recent clinical trials for the National Cholesterol Education Program Adult Treatment Panel III guidelines. *Circulation* 2004;110:227–239

48. Stone NJ, Robinson JG, Lichtenstein AH, et al. 2013 ACC/AHA guideline on the treatment of blood cholesterol to reduce atherosclerotic cardiovascular risk in adults: a report of the American College of Cardiology/American Heart Association Task Force on Practice Guidelines. *Circulation* 2014;129(25 Suppl. 2):S1–S45

49. American Diabetes Association. Cardiovascular disease and risk management. *Diabetes Care* 2016;39(Suppl. 1):S60–S71

50. Gotto AM Jr. Jeremiah Metzger Lecture: cholesterol, inflammation and atherosclerotic cardiovascular disease: is it all LDL? *Trans Am Clin Climatol Assoc* 2011;122:256–289

51. Waters DD, Brotons C, Chiang CW, et al. Lipid Treatment Assessment Project 2: a multinational survey to evaluate the proportion of patients achieving low-density lipoprotein cholesterol goals. *Circulation* 2009;120:28–34

52. Cannon CP, Blazing MA, Giugliano RP, et al. Ezetimibe added to statin therapy after acute coronary syndromes. *N Engl J Med* 2015;372:2387–2397

53. Miller M, Stone NJ, Ballantyne C, et al. Triglycerides and cardiovascular disease: a scientific statement from the American Heart Association. *Circulation* 2011;123:2292–2333

54. Frick MH, Elo O, Haapa K, et al. Helsinki Heart Study: primary-prevention trial with gemfibrozil in middle-aged men with dyslipidemia: safety of treatment, changes in risk factors, and incidence of coronary heart disease. *N Engl J Med* 1987;317:1237–1245

55. Rubins HB, Robins SJ, Collins D, et al.; Veterans Affairs High-Density Lipoprotein Cholesterol Intervention Trial Study Group. Gemfibrozil for the secondary prevention of coronary heart disease in men with low levels of high-density lipoprotein cholesterol. *N Engl J Med* 1999;341:410–418

56. Jun M, Foote C, Lv J, et al. Effects of fibrates on cardiovascular outcomes: a systematic review and meta-analysis. *Lancet* 2010;375:1875–1884

57. Wierzbicki AS, Mikhailidis DP, Wray R, et al. Statin-fibrate combination: therapy for hyperlipidemia: a review. *Curr Med Res Opin* 2003;19:155–168

58. Jones PH, Davidson MH. Reporting rate of rhabdomyolysis with fenofibrate + statin versus gemfibrozil + any statin. *Am J Cardiol* 2005;95:120–122

59. Ginsberg HN, Elam MB, Lovato LC, et al. Effects of combination lipid therapy in type 2 diabetes mellitus. *N Engl J Med* 2010;362:1563–1574

60. American Diabetes Association. Microvascular complications and foot care. *Diabetes Care* 2016;39(Suppl. 1):S72–S80

61. Lewis EJ, Hunsicker LG, Bain RP, Rohde RD, the Collaborative Study Group. The effect of angiotensin-converting-enzyme inhibition on diabetic nephropathy. *N Engl J Med* 1993;329:1456–1462

62. Brenner BM, Cooper ME, de Zeeuw D, et al. Effects of losartan on renal and cardiovascular outcomes in patients with type 2 diabetes and nephropathy. *N Engl J Med* 2001;345:861–869

63. Lewis EJ, Hunsicker LG, Clarke WR, et al. Renoprotective effect of the angiotensin-receptor antagonist irbesartan in patients with nephropathy due to type 2 diabetes. *N Engl J Med* 2001;345:851–860

64. Strippoli GF, Craig M, Deeks JJ, Schena FP, Craig JC. Effects of angiotensin converting enzyme inhibitors and angiotensin II receptor antagonists on mortality and renal outcomes in diabetic nephropathy: systematic review. *BMJ* 2004;329:828

65. Vejakama P, Thakkinstian A, Lertrattananon D, Ingsathit A, Ngarmukos C, Attia J. Reno-protective effects of renin-angiotensin system blockade in type 2 diabetic patients: a systematic review and network meta-analysis. *Diabetologia* 2012;55:566–578

66. Wu HY, Huang JW, Lin HJ, et al. Comparative effectiveness of renin-angiotensin system blockers and other antihypertensive drugs in patients with diabetes: systematic review and Bayesian network meta-analysis. *BMJ* 2013;347:f6008

67. Dusing R, Sellers F. ACE inhibitors, angiotensin receptor blockers and direct renin inhibitors in combination: a review of their role after the ONTARGET trial. *Curr Med Res Opin* 2009;25:2287–2301

68. Laffel LM, McGill JB, Gans DJ, North American Microalbuminuria Study Group. The beneficial effect of angiotensin-converting enzyme inhibition with captopril on diabetic nephropathy in normotensive IDDM patients with microalbuminuria. *Am J Med* 1995;9:497–504

69. Ravid M, Savin H, Jutrin I, et al. Long-term stabilizing effect of angiotensin-converting enzyme inhibition on plasma creatinine and on proteinuria in normotensive type II diabetic patients. *Ann Intern Med* 1993;118:577–581

70. Ravid M, Lang R, Rachmani R, Lishner M. Long-term renoprotective effect of angiotensin-converting enzyme inhibition in non-insulin-dependent diabetes mellitus: a 7-year follow-up study. *Arch Intern Med* 1996;156:286–289

71. Kasiske BL, Kalil RS, Ma JZ, Liao M, Keane WF. Effect of antihypertensive therapy on the kidney in patients with diabetes: a meta-regression analysis. *Ann Intern Med* 1993;118:129–138

72. Bilous R, Chaturvedi N, Sjolie AK, et al. Effect of candesartan on microalbuminuria and albumin excretion rate in diabetes: three randomized trials. *Ann Intern Med* 2009;151:11–20

73. Curb JD, Pressel SL, Cutler JA, et al.; Systolic Hypertension in the Elderly Program Cooperative Research Group. Effect of diuretic-based antihypertensive treatment on cardiovascular disease risk in older diabetic patients with isolated systolic hypertension. *JAMA* 1996;276:1886–1892

74. Tuomilehto J, Rastenyte D, Birkenhager WH, et al.; Systolic Hypertension in Europe Trial Investigators. Effects of calcium-channel blockade in older patients with diabetes and systolic hypertension. *N Engl J Med* 1999;340:677–684

75. UK Prospective Diabetes Study Group. Tight blood pressure control and risk of macrovascular and microvascular complications in type 2 diabetes: UKPDS 38. *BMJ* 1998;317:703–713

76. Hansson L, Zanchetti A, Carruthers SG, et al.; HOT Study Group. Effects of intensive blood-pressure lowering and low-dose aspirin in patients with hypertension: principal results of the Hypertension Optimal Treatment (HOT) randomised trial. *Lancet* 1998;351:1755–1762

77. Estacio RO, Jeffers BW, Gifford N, Schrier RW. Effect of blood pressure control on diabetic microvascular complications in patients with hypertension and type 2 diabetes. *Diabetes Care* 2000;23(Suppl. 2):B54–B64

78. Lewington S, Clarke R, Qizilbash N, Peto R, Collins R. Age-specific relevance of usual blood pressure to vascular mortality: a meta-analysis of individual data for one million adults in 61 prospective studies. *Lancet* 2002;360:1903–1913

79. Cushman WC, Evans GW, Byington RP, et al. Effects of intensive blood-pressure control in type 2 diabetes mellitus. *N Engl J Med* 2010;362:1575–1585

80. Patel A, MacMahon S, Chalmers J, et al. Effects of a fixed combination of perindopril and indapamide on macrovascular and microvascular outcomes in patients with type 2 diabetes mellitus (the ADVANCE trial): a randomised controlled trial. *Lancet* 2007;370:829–840

81. Zoungas S, Chalmers J, Neal B, et al. Follow-up of blood-pressure lowering and glucose control in type 2 diabetes. *N Engl J Med* 2014;371:1392–1406

82. McBrien K, Rabi DM, Campbell N, et al. Intensive and standard blood pressure targets in patients with type 2 diabetes mellitus: systematic review and meta-analysis. *Arch Intern Med* 2012;172:1296–1303

83. Arguedas JA, Leiva V, Wright JM. Blood pressure targets for hypertension in people with diabetes mellitus. *Cochrane Database Syst Rev* 2013;10:CD008277

84. James PA, Oparil S, Carter BL, et al. 2014 evidence-based guideline for the management of high blood pressure in adults: report from the panel members appointed to the Eighth Joint National Committee (JNC 8). *JAMA* 2014;311:507–520

85. Holman RR, Paul SK, Bethel MA, Neil HA, Matthews DR. Long-term follow-up after tight control of blood pressure in type 2 diabetes. *N Engl J Med* 2008;359:1565–1576

86. Parving HH, Andersen AR, Smidt UM, et al. Effect of antihypertensive treatment on kidney function in diabetic nephropathy. *Br Med J (Clin Res Ed)* 1987;294:1443–1447

87. Diabetic Retinopathy Study Research Group. Photocoagulation treatment of proliferative diabetic retinopathy: clinical application of Diabetic Retinopathy Study (DRS) findings, DRS Report Number 8. *Ophthalmology* 1981;88:583–600.

88. Early Treatment Diabetic Retinopathy Study Research Group. Photocoagulation for diabetic macular edema: Early Treatment Diabetic Retinopathy Study report number 1. *Arch Ophthalmol* 1985;103:1796–1806

89. Gupta N, Mansoor S, Sharma A, et al. Diabetic retinopathy and VEGF. *Open Ophthalmol J* 2013;7:4–10

90. Agardh E, Tababat-Khani P. Adopting 3-year screening intervals for sight-threatening retinal vascular lesions in type 2 diabetic subjects without retinopathy. *Diabetes Care* 2011;34:1318–1319

91. Peters AL, Davidson MB, Ziel FH. Cost-effective screening for diabetic retinopathy using a nonmydriatic retinal camera in a prepaid health-care setting. *Diabetes Care* 1993;16:1193–1195

92. Germain N, Galusca B, Deb-Joardar N, et al. No loss of chance of diabetic retinopathy screening by endocrinologists with a digital fundus camera. *Diabetes Care* 2011;34:580–585

93. Singh N, Armstrong DG, Lipsky BA. Preventing foot ulcers in patients with diabetes. *JAMA* 2005;293:217–228

94. Boyko EJ, Ahroni JH, Stensel V, et al. A prospective study of risk factors for diabetic foot ulcer: the Seattle Diabetic Foot Study. *Diabetes Care* 1999;22:1036–1042

95. Pham H, Armstrong DG, Harvey C, et al. Screening techniques to identify people at high risk for diabetic foot ulceration: a prospective multicenter trial. *Diabetes Care* 2000;23:606–611

96. Li Y, Burrows NR, Gregg EW, et al. Declining rates of hospitalization for nontraumatic lower-extremity amputation in the diabetic population aged 40 years or older: U.S., 1988–2008. *Diabetes Care* 2012;35:273–277

97. ETDRS Investigators. Aspirin effects on mortality and morbidity in patients with diabetes mellitus: Early Treatment Diabetic Retinopathy Study report 14. *JAMA* 1992;268:1292–1300

98. Ogawa H, Nakayama M, Morimoto T, et al. Low-dose aspirin for primary prevention of atherosclerotic events in patients with type 2 diabetes: a randomized controlled trial. *JAMA* 2008;300:2134–2141

99. Belch J, MacCuish A, Campbell I, et al. The Prevention of Progression of Arterial Disease and Diabetes (POPADAD) Trial: factorial randomised placebo controlled trial of aspirin and antioxidants in patients with diabetes and asymptomatic peripheral arterial disease. *BMJ* 2008;337:a1840

100. Antithrombotic Trialists' Collaboration. Collaborative meta-analysis of randomised trials of antiplatelet therapy for prevention of death, myocardial infarction, and stroke in high risk patients. *BMJ* 2002;324:71–86

101. Baigent C, Blackwell L, Collins R, et al. Aspirin in the primary and secondary prevention of vascular disease: collaborative meta-analysis of individual participant data from randomised trials. *Lancet* 2009;373:1849–1860

102. Kelly JP, Kaufman DW, Jurgelon JM, et al. Risk of aspirin-associated major upper-gastrointestinal bleeding with enteric-coated or buffered product. *Lancet* 1996;348:1413–1416

103. Bhatt DL, Marso SP, Hirsch AT, et al. Amplified benefit of clopidogrel versus aspirin in patients with diabetes mellitus. *Am J Cardiol* 2002;90:625–628

104. CAPRIE Steering Committee. A randomised, blinded, trial of clopidogrel versus aspirin in patients at risk of ischaemic events (CAPRIE). *Lancet* 1996;348:1329–1339

105. Jamal A, Agaku IT, O'Connor E, et al. Current cigarette smoking among adults: United States, 2005–2013. *MMWR* 2014;63:1108–1112.

106. Haire-Joshu D, Glasgow RE, Tibbs TL. Smoking and diabetes. *Diabetes Care* 1999;22:1887–1898

107. Jamal A, Dube SR, Malarcher AM, Shaw L, Engstrom MC. Tobacco use screening and counseling during physician office visits among adults: National Ambulatory Medical Care Survey and National Health Interview Survey, United States, 2005–2009. *MMWR* 2012;61(Suppl.):38–45

108. Chiolero A, Faeh D, Paccaud F, Cornuz J. Consequences of smoking for body weight, body fat distribution, and insulin resistance. *Am J Clin Nutr* 2008;87:801–809

109. Gerber PA, Locher R, Schmid B, et al. Smoking is associated with impaired long-term glucose metabolism in patients with type 1 diabetes mellitus. *Nutr Metab Cardiovasc Dis* 2013;23:102–108

110. Chase HP, Garg SK, Marshall G, et al. Cigarette smoking increases the risk of albuminuria among subjects with type I diabetes. *JAMA* 1991;265:614–617

111. Sands ML, Shetterly SM, Franklin GM, Hamman RF. Incidence of distal symmetric (sensory) neuropathy in NIDDM: the San Luis Valley Diabetes Study. *Diabetes Care* 1997;20:322–329

112. Gunton JE, Davies L, Wilmshurst E, et al. Cigarette smoking affects glycemic control in diabetes. *Diabetes Care* 2002;25:796–797

113. Voulgari C, Katsilambros N, Tentolouris N. Smoking cessation predicts amelioration of microalbuminuria in newly diagnosed type 2 diabetes mellitus: a 1-year prospective study. *Metab Clin Exp* 2011;60:1456–1464

114. Filozof C, Fernandez Pinilla MC, Fernandez-Cruz A. Smoking cessation and weight gain. *Obes Rev* 2004;5:95–103

115. Parsons AC, Shraim M, Inglis J, Aveyard P, Hajek P. Interventions for preventing weight gain after smoking cessation. *Cochrane Database Syst Rev* 2009:CD006219

116. Clair C, Rigotti NA, Porneala B, et al. Association of smoking cessation and weight change with cardiovascular disease among adults with and without diabetes. *JAMA* 2013;309:1014–1021

117. American Diabetes Association. Foundations of care and comprehensive medical evaluation. *Diabetes Care* 2016;39(Suppl 1):S23-S35.

118. Ackermann RT, Thompson TJ, Selby JV, et al. Is the number of documented diabetes process-of-care indicators associated with cardiometabolic risk factor levels, patient satisfaction, or self-rated quality of diabetes care? The Translating Research into Action for Diabetes (TRIAD) Study. *Diabetes Care* 2006;29:2108–2113

119. Mangione CM, Gerzoff RB, Williamson DF, et al. The association between quality of care and the intensity of diabetes disease management programs. *Ann Intern Med* 2006;145:107–116

120. Stark Casagrande S, Fradkin JE, Saydah SH, Rust KF, Cowie CC. The prevalence of meeting A1C, blood pressure, and LDL goals among people with diabetes, 1988–2010. *Diabetes Care* 2013;36:2271–2279

121. Rosen AB. Indications for and utilization of ACE inhibitors in older individuals with diabetes: findings from the National Health and Nutrition Examination Survey 1999 to 2002. *J Gen Intern Med* 2006;21:315–319

122. Fan AZ, Rock V, Zhang X, et al. Trends in cigarette smoking rates and quit attempts among adults with and without diagnosed diabetes, United States, 2001–2010. *Prev Chronic Dis* 2013;10:E160

123. Akers MF, Lutfiyya MN, Amaro ML, Swanoski MT. Prevalence of daily or near daily aspirin use by US adults with diabetes: a cross-sectional study using a multi-year national database. *Health* 2012;4:297–303

124. U.S. Department of Health and Human Services, Centers for Disease Control and Prevention. *Diabetes Report Card 2012.* Atlanta, GA, Centers for Disease Control and Prevention, 2012

125. Turchin A, Shubina M, Pendergrass ML. Relationship of physician volume with process measures and outcomes in diabetes. *Diabetes Care* 2007;30:1442–1447

126. Parchman ML, Pugh JA, Romero RL, Bowers KW. Competing demands or clinical inertia: the case of elevated glycosylated hemoglobin. *Ann Fam Med* 2007;5:196–201

127. Brown JB, Nichols GA. Slow response to loss of glycemic control in type 2 diabetes mellitus. *Am J Manag Care* 2003;9:213–217

128. Brown JB, Nichols GA, Perry A. The burden of treatment failure in type 2 diabetes. *Diabetes Care* 2004;27:1535–1540

129. Nichols GA, Koo YH, Shah SN. Delay of insulin addition to oral combination therapy despite inadequate glycemic control: delay of insulin therapy. *J Gen Intern Med* 2007;22:453–458

130. Rubino A, McQuay LJ, Gough SC, et al. Delayed initiation of subcutaneous insulin therapy after failure of oral glucose-lowering agents in patients with type 2 diabetes: a population-based analysis in the UK. *Diabet Med* 2007;24:1412–1418

131. Khunti K, Wolden ML, Thorsted BL, et al. Clinical inertia in people with type 2 diabetes: a retrospective cohort study of more than 80,000 people. *Diabetes Care* 2013;36:3411–3417

132. Shah BR, Hux JE, Laupacis A, et al. Clinical inertia in response to inadequate glycemic control: do specialists differ from primary care physicians? *Diabetes Care* 2005;28:600–606

133. Braga M, Casanova A, Teoh H, et al. Treatment gaps in the management of cardiovascular risk factors in patients with type 2 diabetes in Canada. *Can J Cardiol* 2010;26:297–302

134. Grant RW, Buse JB, Meigs JB. Quality of diabetes care in U.S. academic medical centers: low rates of medical regimen change. *Diabetes Care* 2005;28:337–442

135. Aujoulat I, Jacquemin P, Rietzschel E, et al. Factors associated with clinical inertia: an integrative review. *Adv Med Educ Pract* 2014;5:141–147

136. Davidson MB, Castellanos M, Duran P, Karlan V. Effective diabetes care by a registered nurse following treatment algorithms in a minority population. *Am J Manag Care* 2006;12:226–232

137. Davidson MB, Blanco-Castellanos M, Duran P. Integrating nurse-directed diabetes management into a primary care setting. *Am J Manag Care* 2010;16:652–656

Chapter 2
Evidence-Based Principles of Nonpharmacological Therapy

DIABETES SELF-MANAGEMENT EDUCATION AND SUPPORT (DSME/DSMS)

Although long recognized as a cornerstone of diabetes management, evidence supporting the benefits of nonpharmacological interventions for glycemic control has emerged only in recent years. Although much of the evidence in this area consists of small, low-quality studies and widely heterogeneous interventions, there is some clinical trial evidence that these interventions improve clinically important outcomes. It should be noted that in any trial, an outcome measure needs to achieve not only *statistical* significance to indicate that the effect was likely real, but also *clinical* significance, i.e., the size of the effect should be sufficiently meaningful for patient care. With respect to lowering of A1C, the U.S. Food and Drug Administration uses an arbitrary threshold of a 0.3–0.4% change as a "non-inferiority" margin.[1] Therefore, while treatment effects at or below this magnitude may be reported as statistically significant, the clinical significance of such modest effects for patient care may be debatable.

An important part of optimal diabetes management is diabetes self-management education (DSME) and diabetes self-management support (DSMS). DSME is the ongoing process of facilitating the knowledge, skills, and abilities necessary for optimal diabetes self-care.[2] DSMS includes activities that assist people with diabetes in implementing and sustaining the behaviors needed to manage their condition on an ongoing basis.[2] These strategies are intended to facilitate patients' own problem-solving and informed decision-making abilities and to foster an ongoing, active collaboration with the patient's health care provider team. The American Diabetes Association (ADA) recommends DSME/DSMS for all patients with diabetes.[3] However, much of the literature on DSME yields mixed findings. In type 2 diabetes, one meta-analysis of 31 randomized controlled trials of DSME interventions found that glycohemoglobin levels were reduced by 0.76% compared to controls immediately after the conclusion of the DSME program. The meta-analysis also found that greater contact time with the diabetes educator correlated with a better outcome, but the magnitude of reduction fell to only 0.26% versus controls with another 1–3 months of follow-up.[4] A more recent meta-analysis of 21 randomized controlled trials in type 2 diabetes found a mean A1C reduction of 0.44% at 6 months.[5] In contrast, other studies of empowerment-based DSME programs compared to usual care either failed to show any effect on lowering A1C[6–8] or found A1C lowering that was indistinguishable from that of usual care.[9,10] Significant quality-of-life improvements were found in a meta-analysis of 20 DSME intervention studies involving 1,892 patients with type 1 or type 2 diabetes,[11] while other studies reported improvements in other surrogate behavioral measures such as self-management knowledge and skills,[5] self-efficacy,[5] and diabetes distresss.[12] DSME may also be associated with fewer hospitalizations and lower health care costs,[13,14] particularly when delivered by trained diabetes educators as part of a formally accredited program.[15] Thus, while there is some value of DSME for improving some important clinical measures, the body of evidence is not consistent or strong. Thus, appropriate and timely treatment with pharmacological agents will still be critically important to optimally improve glucose control.[16]

National standards have been established to define the qualities of DSME/DSMS programs that exemplify effective and excellent education strategies and help to formalize program recognition and accreditation.[2] DSME teaching may be delivered by non-physician allied health professionals who have the appropriate training and should ideally be delivered with a culturally and age-appropriate, patient-focused, empowerment- and skills-based approach, encompassing aspects of psychosocial and emotional support. DSME teaching should not simply be a didactic delivery of information to the patient. The ADA, the American Association of Diabetes Educators (AADE), and the Academy of Nutrition and Dietetics jointly recommend that DSME should be considered, provided, and/or adjusted for all type 2 diabetic patients at the following times: *1)* upon initial diagnosis, *2)* repeated annually, *3)* whenever new complicating factors develop (e.g., new-onset complications or comorbidities that might complicate self-management), and *4)* when transitions in care occur (e.g., a new health care setting or team, new transitions in living situations).[17] Whether DSME can actually be provided at all of these times will depend on local resources or reimbursements. At our institution, as a minimum, all newly diagnosed and newly referred patients are referred to a group DSME class administered by a certified diabetes educator (CDE), as well as any patients needing to update their knowledge or skills after a prolonged absence or lapse in care.

MEDICAL NUTRITION THERAPY

Optimizing nutrition is critical for all patients with diabetes.[3] However, nutrition management is inherently complex and particularly so for patients with diabetes who must pay attention to multiple factors in proper meal planning. Medical nutrition therapy (MNT) refers to the individualized nutrition planning for diabetes that is administered by health care professionals who are familiar with its principles and practice, such as registered dietitians or appropriately trained CDEs, with an intent to improve overall health, achieve the patient's metabolic goals, and delay diabetes complications. Much of the literature on the benefits of the various aspects of MNT includes mixed findings because of factors such as heterogeneous study methodologies, mixed effects any time macronutrient changes are made, inaccurate measurement of actual dietary intake, lack of proper blinding, and confounding by concurrent weight and/or medication changes.

However, the ADA still bases many of its recommendations on the available evidence, much of which is supportive.

Given the complexity of MNT, the wide heterogeneity of different cultures and lifestyle practices, and substantial intra- and interindividual variability in the implementation and responses to nutritional interventions, it is now accepted that there is no "ideal" nutritional regimen that is applicable for all diabetic patients. Instead, MNT should be individualized for each patient's unique needs, personal and cultural preferences, and metabolic goals.[3,18] However, all eating patterns should emphasize an appropriate total caloric intake and a balance of macronutrients and micronutrients from healthy sources, which may be exemplified by certain eating patterns. For example, while "Mediterranean-style" meal patterns may be loosely defined and highly variable, some studies have found that they can improve glucose and lipid control compared to usual diets.[19,20] The PREDIMED study showed that such a dietary pattern can reduce cardiovascular events compared to a control diet.[21] The Dietary Approaches to Stop Hypertension (DASH) method has been shown to reduce A1C, lipids, and blood pressure (BP) compared to a control diet in type 2 diabetic patients.[22] Plant-based (vegetarian or vegan) approaches have also been shown to lower weight and A1C in diabetic patients.[23] Successful self-implementation of any recommended eating pattern is a longitudinal and progressive learning process for most patients, often requiring sustained educational support and feedback. Thus, in drug-naive patients, initiation of pharmacological therapy should not be delayed, and more intensive MNT teaching should be considered whenever it is practical in patients who are inadequately controlled with pharmacotherapy.[24]

A comprehensive review of MNT teaching is beyond the scope of this chapter, but some of its major principles and supporting evidence will be briefly discussed.

TOTAL CALORIES AND WEIGHT CONTROL

Overweight or obese diabetic patients should be prescribed a calorie-reducing dietary plan to facilitate weight loss, while still maintaining a healthy eating pattern. Although a recent meta-analysis found most weight loss trials in patients with type 2 diabetes produced <5% weight loss and no significant overall glycemic benefit,[25] studies that do achieve 5–8% weight loss, well below the degree of weight loss desired by most individuals, are capable of producing substantial metabolic benefits. For example, a trial using prepared meal plans in patients with type 2 diabetes that produced a mere 6% weight loss (compared to 2% with usual care) after 6 months resulted in A1C improvements of 0.87% and 0.22%, respectively; lipids and BP also improved.[26] A Mediterranean diet in newly diagnosed, treatment-naive patients with type 2 diabetes produced a 7.2% and 4.4% weight loss from baseline in the first and fourth years, respectively, and they had a respective 1.2% and 0.9% reduction in A1C from baseline, both significantly greater than the comparison low-fat diet, which produced a respective 4.9% and 3.7% weight loss and a 0.6% and 0.5% A1C reduction. In this study, lipids and BP also improved, and there was comparatively less need for anti-hyperglycemic medications at both 18 months and 4 years.[19] The landmark Look AHEAD study found that an intensive lifestyle modification weight loss program, at least over the first year, that produced 8.6% weight loss reduced A1C from 7.3% to 6.6% (0.7%

reduction), compared to only 0.7% weight loss and an A1C drop from 7.3% to only 7.2% using routine education and support. Lipids, BP, albuminuria, and need for anti-hyperglycemic medications all improved significantly with intensive lifestyle modification in this study as well.[27] When indicated, adjunctive weight loss enhancements, such as anti-obesity medications[28-31] or particularly bariatric surgery,[32,33] which can reduce hyperglycemia in the short-term independent of any weight loss,[34] may also be helpful.[35] However, adherence to MNT should always remain the focus of any long-term weight-control efforts.[36]

Regardless of the means by which weight loss is achieved, improvements are almost always more pronounced in the shorter term (e.g., within 6–12 months), while sustained weight loss compared to controls beyond 12 months either becomes less pronounced with longer follow-up or the lost weight is completely regained.[37,38] For example, after 9.6 years of follow-up in the Look AHEAD trial, progressive weight regain substantially narrowed the benefit between intensive treatment and controls.[39] Even with the potent effects of bariatric surgery, there is a gradual weight regain with follow-up for several years after the initial weight loss.[32] Thus, long-term efforts to sustain the initial caloric deficit can be particularly challenging, but are clearly important.

Both dietary fat and carbohydrates contribute to energy balance. Although dietary fat (at 9 kcal per gram) is more energy dense than carbohydrates (4 kcal per gram), dietary fat restriction without preventing a compensatory increase in dietary carbohydrates will not be as effective for weight loss as dietary plans that limit both macronutrients. In the short-term, carbohydrate restriction may produce comparatively greater weight loss than dietary fat restriction,[40,41] in part because of an initial diuresis that accompanies acute carbohydrate restriction (and not an actual loss of fat mass).[42] But with longer follow-up, there are essentially no differences in weight loss efficacy between fat restriction and carbohydrate restriction strategies.[41-43]

Estimating a patient's dietary caloric requirements is an important part of proper MNT meal planning. Gold standard methods to measure a person's energy requirements are usually too cumbersome or require specialized equipment, but several estimation methods exist (with varying degrees of accuracy for obese individuals).[44] Table 2.1 summarizes one such method for sedentary individuals, based on desirable body weight in relation to height and body frame size, which we use in our diabetes clinic.[45] Physicians who may not be familiar with MNT can also easily use this method as part of their MNT referral.

DIETARY CARBOHYDRATES

Carbohydrates are the most important dietary contributor to daily variations in glucose, so their control should be a major focus,[46] particularly for insulin-treated patients taking a prandial (i.e., short- or rapid-acting) insulin formulation. Carbohydrates are also a major determinant of weight control, since they typically comprise the largest proportion of total daily calories (averaging ~45–50%).[47,48] Excessive carbohydrate intake can also exacerbate dyslipidemia and cardio-metabolic risk (specifically, higher triglycerides and lower HDL cholesterol).[49]

The ADA recommends that insulin-treated patients capable of following an intensive, flexible insulin regimen (such as many patients with type 1 diabetes)

Table 2.1. Calculating Patients' Dietary Caloric Needs

1. Estimate desirable body weight (DBW)		

a. Height	Females	Males
For the first 5 ft:	100 lb	106 lb
Each inch over 5 ft:	5 lb	6 lb

b. Frame size: 10% is added to the DBW for large-framed individuals, and 10% is subtracted for small-framed subjects. Frame size can be estimated by having the patient's dominant hand grasp the other wrist and oppose the thumb and middle finger. If these two fingers meet, the patient has a medium frame (and no DBW adjustment is necessary). If they overlap appreciably, the patient is small framed. If they fail to meet, the patient is large framed. Appropriate adjustments are made to the DBW in the latter two circumstances. Patients who are ≥120% of DBW (i.e., ≥20% over their DBW) are considered overweight or obese, and patients <120% of DBW are considered lean.

2. Calculate calorie content

To lose weight: 10 calories per lb of DBW
To maintain weight: 15 calories per lb of DBW
To gain weight: 20 calories per lb of DBW
Lower limit: 1,000 calories

3. Adjust for age (since basal metabolic rate decreases with increasing age)

<50 years: No change
50–60 years: Subtract 10% from calorie content, if sedentary
>60 years: Subtract 20% from calorie content, if sedentary
Lower limit: 1,000 calories

should be taught a variable carbohydrate-counting approach to meal planning,[3] which can improve their glucose control compared to usual care.[50] One study comparing this approach to empiric prandial insulin dose adjustments in patients with type 1 diabetes found that A1C was 0.35% lower after discounting those subjects who were inconsistent with performing carbohydrate counting.[51] However, another study comparing carbohydrate counting to a strategy that did not use carbohydrate counting in type 2 diabetic patients failed to find a significant A1C advantage.[52] Insulin-treated patients who are not following a flexible insulin regimen or performing carbohydrate counting but are following a fixed-dose insulin regimen should be taught to adopt consistent daily carbohydrate intakes (e.g., using a carbohydrate exchange approach or experience-based estimation).[3] The ADA also recommends that any patient with diabetes with learning or health literacy barriers that make learning such skills difficult should at least follow a simpler meal-planning approach (e.g., attention to portion control and making generally healthful food choices).[3,53]

As to food choices among different types of carbohydrate sources, whole grains, vegetables and fruits, legumes, and dairy sources should be emphasized over choices that are rich in simple sugars, added fats, or sodium.[3] There is actually limited clinical trial evidence supporting the glycemic benefits of these specific nutrients, although whole grains may help lower glucose because of their fiber content.[54] Legumes, as part of a dietary plan with foods that have a low glycemic index (GI, defined as the postprandial absorption pattern of a single carbohydrate food), may lower A1C more than whole grains.[55] Foods rich in dietary fiber should be encouraged, but more for their favorable effect on cardiovascular risk factors[56,57] than actual A1C lowering. The GI of any carbohydrate food is highly sensitive to the exact form of the food (e.g., a whole apple versus applesauce versus apple juice) and its nutrient context (e.g., bread eaten alone versus with a sandwich); but meal plans with lower-GI foods (i.e., a more gradual absorption pattern) may be associated with an improvement in A1C of about 0.5% compared to meal plans with higher-GI foods.[58] However, GI should not be confused with glycemic load (i.e., the actual quantity of carbohydrate ingested), which may be a more important determinant of glucose control.[59] Vegetables, fruits, and dairy foods are not supported by clinical trial evidence for glucose lowering, but prospective cohort studies suggest that they may benefit weight control and cardiovascular risk.[57,60,61] Sugar-sweetened beverages (such as those containing high-fructose corn syrup), according to cohort studies,[62–64] may contribute to obesity and worsen cardio-metabolic risk and should be completely avoided if possible. While *occasional* isocaloric substitution of healthier carbohydrates with sucrose-containing foods (sweets) may not worsen glucose control,[65] it should be minimized.

DIETARY FAT

Because dyslipidemia and cardiovascular risk often accompany diabetes (particularly type 2 diabetes), control of dietary fat is also important for diabetic patients. As for the general population, dietary fat should ideally encompass between 20 and 35% of total daily calories for diabetic patients; the actual percentage should be individualized.[3] As to choices among different types of dietary fats, foods high in saturated and *trans* fats can elevate LDL cholesterol levels,[66] so foods rich in polyunsaturated or monounsaturated fat sources are preferred, since they may lower LDL cholesterol levels.[66] In one study with diabetic patients, dietary enrichment with monounsaturated fats reduced A1C by 0.8% compared to a conventional diet, although the proportion of dietary carbohydrates was also lower.[67] Before the widespread use of HMG-CoA reductase inhibitors (statins), some studies supported a cardiovascular benefit of modest intake of marine, long-chain omega-3 fatty acids (specifically, eicosapentaenoic acid [EPA] and docosahexaenoic acid [DHA]),[68] particularly through eating fatty fish; at least two servings per week is still recommended.[3] However, glycemic benefits have never been shown in diabetic patients, and the recent Outcome Reduction with an Initial Glargine Intervention (ORIGIN) trial of prediabetic and diabetic patients given omega-3 fish oils versus olive oil (53% of whom were already taking statins) failed to show any cardiovascular benefit.[69] Higher doses of these two marine fish oils (total of 3–4 g/day) may lower triglycerides, but the cardiovascular benefits of this strategy in diabetic patients remain unclear.[68]

DIETARY PROTEIN

Dietary protein is an obligatory macronutrient that should not normally be used for energy needs. It typically comprises ~15–20% of total daily calories, although the actual amount should be individualized.[3] Increasing protein as a means to reduce the carbohydrate proportion without increasing dietary fat can lead to short-term glycemic improvements.[70,71] For patients with diabetic nephropathy, restriction of dietary protein below the recommended daily allowance of 0.8 g/kg/day does not meaningfully reduce glycemia, nephropathy progression, or cardio-metabolic risk and is therefore not necessary.[72,73] There is scant literature on the benefits of different sources of protein in diabetic individuals, except possible favorable effects of dietary soy protein compared to animal protein on lipids and markers of nephropathy.[74,75] One study of soy phytoestrogen supplements showed a minimal (although statistically significant) 0.1% A1C reduction compared to blinded placebo (but this is of questionable clinical significance), along with a small (12%) lowering of LDL cholesterol.[76]

OVERALL MACRONUTRIENT COMPOSITION

Notwithstanding the foregoing discussions of individual macronutrients (dietary carbohydrates, fat, and protein), it should be emphasized again that studies that have directly compared diets with different macronutrient compositions (carbohydrate content between 35 and 65%, fat content between 20 and 40%, and protein content between 15 and 25%) have not shown any significant differences in their effects on weight loss.[25,43] Only a hypocaloric diet, and not the specific macronutrient composition, can have a positive impact on weight loss.

MICRONUTRIENTS, ALCOHOL, AND DIETARY SUPPLEMENTS

Dietary sodium is the most important mineral for diabetic patients because of its influence on BP and cardiovascular risk; reducing excess dietary sodium effectively reduces BP.[77] The ADA currently recommends that all diabetic patients consume no more than 2,300 mg sodium daily.[3] For diabetic patients with coexisting hypertension, further restriction to <1,500 mg daily will produce greater BP lowering, but prospective follow-up studies suggest that such intensive reduction may not be associated with further reductions in adverse outcomes.[78,79] They also may not be easily achievable for some because of limited availability and/or palatability of low-sodium food choices while still maintaining a nutritionally adequate diet.[80] Thus, any such stringent dietary sodium restriction should be individualized.

Despite many claims as to the benefits of other micronutrients, such as chromium, magnesium, vitamin D, or antioxidants (including vitamins C and E), there is inconsistent clinical trial evidence that they have any clinically significant benefits for diabetic patients who are not deficient in these micronutrients[81]; their routine supplementation is therefore not recommended.

The current recommendation for alcohol use is the same as that for the general population: averaging no more than one standard drink per day for women or two per day for men[3] (with one standard drink being 15 g ethanol, typically contained in 12 oz of beer, 5 oz of wine, or 1.5 oz of distilled spirits). A systematic review of studies of alcohol use found a U-shaped relationship between the degree of alcohol use and diabetes incidence, a tendency for alcohol to lower glucose in patients with established diabetes, lower cardiovascular events associated with moderate alcohol use compared to non-use, and possible worsening of diabetic retinopathy associated with heavy alcohol use.[82] Diabetic patients who use alcohol should be cautioned that ethanol inhibits hepatic glucose output and therefore may predispose to delayed hypoglycemia, particularly for patients taking insulin or insulin secretagogues.[83,84]

There is currently no dietary supplement product (e.g., herbal products or cinnamon) that is supported by consistent, good-quality clinical trial evidence to benefit patients with diabetes.[81]

PHYSICAL ACTIVITY

A regular program of physical activity should be an integral part of all lifestyle modification programs, particularly for overweight or obese patients, where it is an important determinant of long-term prevention of weight regain.[85–87] Weight loss strategies that rely solely on limiting dietary caloric intake often produce a greater degree of weight loss than strategies that rely solely on increasing exercise caloric expenditure.[38] However, solely limiting dietary intake may lead to undesirable loss of lean body (i.e., muscle) mass.[86] Strategies to increase exercise energy expenditure usually produce smaller energy deficits than dietary restriction strategies; very high levels of exercise are capable of achieving a similar energy deficit, but then adherence to the exercise can become a problem.[87] Thus, the two strategies should always complement each other in any weight loss program.

Similar to recommendations for the nondiabetic population, the ADA recommends that diabetic patients engage in at least 150 minutes of moderate-intensity aerobic physical activity per week, spread out over a minimum of 3 days per week, ideally with no more than 2 consecutive days in-between exercise days.[3,88] Moderate intensity is defined as 50–70% of the maximum heart rate (maximum heart rate is calculated as 220 bpm minus the patient's age), which for most people is achievable through activities like walking 1 mile in 15–20 minutes, cycling at 5–9 mph, aerobic dancing or water aerobics, ballroom dancing, or other similar activities.[89] Higher-intensity activities can achieve even greater activity targets or achieve the same goal if performed for less total time, but higher-intensity activities may be harder to do for most diabetic patients. One meta-analysis of exercise trials found that the mean aerobic capacity of typical individuals with diabetes (22.4 mL O_2 consumed per kilogram per minute) would predict that they will experience difficulties maintaining activities such as sweeping, climbing stairs, or many home repair activities.[90] For very sedentary individuals, lower-intensity activities, or even efforts to simply reduce sedentary time or interrupt prolonged sedentary periods (>90 minutes) may confer benefits[3,91]; while not sufficient on their own to meet recommended targets, they can be an important first step in the progression towards adopting higher-intensity activities. Ideally, the aerobic activity program should be complemented with resistance training (e.g., weights) at least twice per week.[88] The combination of an aerobic plus resistance program has been shown to be more beneficial than either approach alone.[92,93]

Even an acute session of exercise can enhance insulin sensitivity and action in a dose-dependent manner; the smaller effect of lower-intensity exercise is detectable with special testing,[94] but its clinical significance is less clear. The physiological effect of a single exercise session lasts at least 24 hours, but less than 72 hours.[88] Regular moderate-intensity physical activity can lower glucose levels in the short term,[88,95] independent of any longer-term weight changes.[96] Numerous studies have documented the glucose-lowering benefits of a regular physical activity program in diabetes,[88,96] with generally greater effects produced by larger exercise doses.[97] Large prospective cohort studies have also documented a strong association between regular physical activity and lower cardiovascular complications and mortality.[98–100]

However, a few caveats apply uniquely to diabetic patients adopting or intensifying physical activity programs. Because physical activity enhances insulin action, patients taking insulin or insulin secretagogues are at risk of exercise-induced hypoglycemia[101] (since their insulin levels are not solely under endogenous control and thus do not fall appropriately in response to falling glucose levels). Such patients, especially if already under good control, should self-monitor their glucose levels before prolonged or vigorous exercise and should be advised to ingest some carbohydrates if the level is already <100 mg/dL.[3,88] Dosages of insulin or insulin secretagogues in these patients may have to be lowered with longer-term maintenance of the exercise program. For patients with type 1 diabetes who are temporarily deprived of insulin for as little as 12–48 hours for any reason, intense exercise should be avoided until insulin is restarted[102]; the acute catecholamine rise of exercise, if unopposed by insulin, can rapidly lead to ketoacidosis.[103] Cardiovascular autonomic neuropathy, which may not be clinically apparent, decreases cardiac responsiveness to exercise and increases the risk of cardiac death and silent myocardial ischemia[104]; therefore, patients with any autonomic neuropathy should ideally undergo cardiac testing before beginning or intensifying an exercise program.[105] In the presence of proliferative or severe non-proliferative retinopathy, *vigorous-intensity* exercise can precipitate retinal hemorrhage or detachment and should be avoided until the high-risk lesions have been treated.[88] Patients with peripheral neuropathy or insensate feet should be cautioned on the importance of proper footwear and to monitor their feet frequently.[88] Although progression of neuropathy may be slowed by regular physical activity,[106] acute foot trauma still remains a risk.

REFERENCES

1. U.S. Department of Health and Human Services, Food and Drug Administration, Center for Drug Evaluation and Research. Guidance for industry. Diabetes mellitus: developing drugs and therapeutic biologics for treatment and prevention, 2008. Available from http://www.fda.gov/downloads/Drugs/.../Guidances/ucm071624.pdf

2. Haas L, Maryniuk M, Beck J, et al. National standards for diabetes self-management education and support. *Diabetes Care* 2012;35:2393–2401

3. American Diabetes Association. Foundations of care and comprehensive medical evaluation. *Diabetes Care* 2016;39(Suppl. 1):S23–S35

4. Norris SL, Lau J, Smith SJ, et al. Self-management education for adults with type 2 diabetes: a meta-analysis of the effect on glycemic control. *Diabetes Care* 2002;25:1159–71

5. Steinsbekk A, Rygg LO, Lisulo M, et al. Group based diabetes self-management education compared to routine treatment for people with type 2 diabetes mellitus: a systematic review with meta-analysis. *BMC Health Serv Res* 2012;12:213

6. Adolfsson ET, Walker-Engstrom ML, Smide B, Wikblad K. Patient education in type 2 diabetes: a randomized controlled 1-year follow-up study. *Diabetes Res Clin Pract* 2007;76:341–350

7. Anderson RM, Funnell MM, Aikens JE, et al. Evaluating the efficacy of an empowerment-based self-management consultant intervention: results of a two-year randomized controlled trial. *Ther Patient Educ* 2009;1:3–11

8. Cooper H, Booth K, Gill G. A trial of empowerment-based education in type 2 diabetes: global rather than glycaemic benefits. *Diabetes Res Clin Pract* 2008;82:165–171

9. Davies MJ, Heller S, Skinner TC, et al. Effectiveness of the diabetes education and self-management for ongoing and newly diagnosed (DESMOND) programme for people with newly diagnosed type 2 diabetes: cluster randomised controlled trial. *BMJ* 2008;336:491–495

10. Khunti K, Gray LJ, Skinner T, et al. Effectiveness of a diabetes education and self-management programme (DESMOND) for people with newly diagnosed type 2 diabetes mellitus: three year follow-up of a cluster randomised controlled trial in primary care. *BMJ* 2012;344:e2333

11. Cochran J, Conn VS. Meta-analysis of quality of life outcomes following diabetes self-management training. *Diabetes Educ* 2008;34:815–823

12. Fisher L, Hessler D, Glasgow RE, et al. REDEEM: a pragmatic trial to reduce diabetes distress. *Diabetes Care* 2013;36:2551–2558

13. Robbins JM, Thatcher GE, Webb DA, Valdmanis VG. Nutritionist visits, diabetes classes, and hospitalization rates and charges: the Urban Diabetes Study. *Diabetes Care* 2008;31:655–660

14. Duncan I, Birkmeyer C, Coughlin S, et al. Assessing the value of diabetes education. *Diabetes Educ* 2009;35:752–760

15. Duncan I, Ahmed T, Li QE, et al. Assessing the value of the diabetes educator. *Diabetes Educ* 2011;37:638–657

16. Davidson MB. How our current medical care system fails people with diabetes: lack of timely, appropriate clinical decisions. *Diabetes Care* 2009;32:370–372

17. Powers MA, Bardsley J, Cypress M, et al. Diabetes self-management education and support in type 2 diabetes: a joint position statement of the American Diabetes Association, the American Association of Diabetes Educators,

and the Academy of Nutrition and Dietetics. *Diabetes Care* 2015;38:1372–1382

18. Wheeler ML, Dunbar SA, Jaacks LM, et al. Macronutrients, food groups, and eating patterns in the management of diabetes: a systematic review of the literature, 2010. *Diabetes Care* 2012;35:434–445

19. Esposito K, Maiorino MI, Ciotola M, et al. Effects of a Mediterranean-style diet on the need for antihyperglycemic drug therapy in patients with newly diagnosed type 2 diabetes: a randomized trial. *Ann Intern Med* 2009;151:306–314

20. Elhayany A, Lustman A, Abel R, et al. A low carbohydrate mediterranean diet improves cardiovascular risk factors and diabetes control among overweight patients with type 2 diabetes mellitus: a 1-year prospective randomized intervention study. *Diabetes Obes Metab* 2010;12:204–209

21. Estruch R, Ros E, Salas-Salvado J, et al. Primary prevention of cardiovascular disease with a Mediterranean diet. *N Engl J Med* 2013;368:1279–1290

22. Azadbakht L, Fard NR, Karimi M, et al. Effects of the Dietary Approaches to Stop Hypertension (DASH) eating plan on cardiovascular risks among type 2 diabetic patients: a randomized crossover clinical trial. *Diabetes Care* 2011;34:55–57

23. Barnard ND, Cohen J, Jenkins DJ, et al. A low-fat vegan diet and a conventional diabetes diet in the treatment of type 2 diabetes: a randomized, controlled, 74-wk clinical trial. *Am J Clin Nutr* 2009;89:1588S–1596S

24. Coppell KJ, Kataoka M, Williams SM, et al. Nutritional intervention in patients with type 2 diabetes who are hyperglycaemic despite optimised drug treatment: Lifestyle Over and Above Drugs in Diabetes (LOADD) study: randomised controlled trial. *BMJ* 2010;341:c3337

25. Franz MJ, Boucher JL, Rutten-Ramos S, VanWormer JJ. Lifestyle weight-loss intervention outcomes in overweight and obese adults with type 2 diabetes: a systematic review and meta-analysis of randomized clinical trials. *J Acad Nutr Diet* 2015;115:1447–1463

26. Metz JA, Stern JS, Kris-Etherton P, et al. A randomized trial of improved weight loss with a prepared meal plan in overweight and obese patients: impact on cardiovascular risk reduction. *Arch Intern Med* 2000;160:2150–2158

27. Pi-Sunyer X, Blackburn G, Brancati FL, et al. Reduction in weight and cardiovascular disease risk factors in individuals with type 2 diabetes: one-year results of the Look AHEAD trial. *Diabetes Care* 2007;30:1374–1383

28. Kelley DE, Bray GA, Pi-Sunyer FX, et al. Clinical efficacy of orlistat therapy in overweight and obese patients with insulin-treated type 2 diabetes: a 1-year randomized controlled trial. *Diabetes Care* 2002;25:1033–1041

29. O'Neil PM, Smith SR, Weissman NJ, et al. Randomized placebo-controlled clinical trial of lorcaserin for weight loss in type 2 diabetes mellitus: the BLOOM-DM study. *Obesity (Silver Spring)* 2012;20:1426–1436

30. Garvey WT, Ryan DH, Bohannon NJ, et al. Weight-loss therapy in type 2 diabetes: effects of phentermine and topiramate extended release. *Diabetes Care* 2014;37:3309–3316

31. Hollander P, Gupta AK, Plodkowski R, et al. Effects of naltrexone sustained-release/bupropion sustained-release combination therapy on body weight and glycemic parameters in overweight and obese patients with type 2 diabetes. *Diabetes Care* 2013;36:4022–4029

32. Sjostrom L, Peltonen M, Jacobson P, et al. Association of bariatric surgery with long-term remission of type 2 diabetes and with microvascular and macrovascular complications. *JAMA* 2014;311:2297–2304

33. Schauer PR, Bhatt DL, Kirwan JP, et al. Bariatric surgery versus intensive medical therapy for diabetes: 3-year outcomes. *N Engl J Med* 2014;370:2002–2013

34. Bradley D, Magkos F, Klein S. Effects of bariatric surgery on glucose homeostasis and type 2 diabetes. *Gastroenterology* 2012;143:897–912

35. American Diabetes Association. Obesity management for the treatment of type 2 diabetes. *Diabetes Care* 2016;39(Suppl. 1):S47–S51

36. American Diabetes Association. Approaches to glycemic treatment. *Diabetes Care* 2016;39(Suppl. 1):S52–S59

37. Dansinger ML, Tatsioni A, Wong JB, et al. Meta-analysis: the effect of dietary counseling for weight loss. *Ann Intern Med* 2007;147:41–50

38. Franz MJ, VanWormer JJ, Crain AL, Boucher JL, Histon T, Caplan W, Bowman JD, Pronk NP. Weight-loss outcomes: a systematic review and meta-analysis of weight-loss clinical trials with a minimum 1-year follow-up. *J Am Diet Assoc* 2007;107:1755–1767

39. Wing RR, Bolin P, Brancati FL, et al. Cardiovascular effects of intensive lifestyle intervention in type 2 diabetes. *N Engl J Med* 2013;369:145–154

40. Bazzano LA, Hu T, Reynolds K, et al. Effects of low-carbohydrate and low-fat diets: a randomized trial. *Ann Intern Med* 2014;161:309–318

41. Davis NJ, Tomuta N, Schechter C, et al. Comparative study of the effects of a 1-year dietary intervention of a low-carbohydrate diet versus a low-fat diet on weight and glycemic control in type 2 diabetes. *Diabetes Care* 2009;32:1147–1152

42. Denke MA. Metabolic effects of high-protein, low-carbohydrate diets. *Am J Cardiol* 2001;88:59–61

43. Sacks FM, Bray GA, Carey VJ, et al. Comparison of weight-loss diets with different compositions of fat, protein, and carbohydrates. *N Engl J Med* 2009;360:859–873

44. de Oliveira EP, Orsatti FL, Teixeira O, et al. Comparison of predictive equations for resting energy expenditure in overweight and obese adults. *J Obes* 2011;2011:534714

45. Hamwi GJ. Therapy: changing dietary concepts. In *Diabetes Mellitus: Diagnosis and Treatment.* Vol 1. Danowski TS, Ed. New York, American Diabetes Association, 1964, p. 73–78

46. Kirk JK, Graves DE, Craven TE, et al. Restricted-carbohydrate diets in patients with type 2 diabetes: a meta-analysis. *J Am Diet Assoc* 2008;108:91–100

47. Eeley EA, Stratton IM, Hadden DR, et al.; UK Prospective Diabetes Study Group. UKPDS 18: estimated dietary intake in type 2 diabetic patients randomly allocated to diet, sulphonylurea or insulin therapy. *Diabet Med* 1996;13:656–662

48. Delahanty LM, Nathan DM, Lachin JM, et al. Association of diet with glycated hemoglobin during intensive treatment of type 1 diabetes in the Diabetes Control and Complications Trial. *Am J Clin Nutr* 2009;89:518–524

49. Parks EJ, Hellerstein MK. Carbohydrate-induced hypertriacylglycerolemia: historical perspective and review of biological mechanisms. *Am J Clin Nutr* 2000;71:412–433

50. DAFNE Study Group. Training in flexible, intensive insulin management to enable dietary freedom in people with type 1 diabetes: dose adjustment for normal eating (DAFNE) randomised controlled trial. *BMJ* 2002;325:746

51. Laurenzi A, Bolla AM, Panigoni G, et al. Effects of carbohydrate counting on glucose control and quality of life over 24 weeks in adult patients with type 1 diabetes on continuous subcutaneous insulin infusion: a randomized, prospective clinical trial (GIOCAR). *Diabetes Care* 2011;34:823–827

52. Bergenstal RM, Johnson M, Powers MA, et al. Adjust to target in type 2 diabetes: comparison of a simple algorithm with carbohydrate counting for adjustment of mealtime insulin glulisine. *Diabetes Care* 2008;31:1305–1310

53. Ziemer DC, Berkowitz KJ, Panayioto RM, et al. A simple meal plan emphasizing healthy food choices is as effective as an exchange-based meal plan for urban African Americans with type 2 diabetes. *Diabetes Care* 2003;26:1719–1724

54. Lu ZX, Walker KZ, Muir JG, O'Dea K. Arabinoxylan fibre improves metabolic control in people with type II diabetes. *Eur J Clin Nutr* 2004;58:621–628

55. Jenkins DJ, Kendall CW, Augustin LS, et al. Effect of legumes as part of a low glycemic index diet on glycemic control and cardiovascular risk factors in type 2 diabetes mellitus: a randomized controlled trial. *Arch Intern Med* 2012;172:1653–1660

56. de Natale C, Annuzzi G, Bozzetto L, et al. Effects of a plant-based high-carbohydrate/high-fiber diet versus high-monounsaturated fat/low-carbohydrate diet on postprandial lipids in type 2 diabetic patients. *Diabetes Care* 2009;32:2168–2173

57. He M, van Dam RM, Rimm E, Hu FB, Qi L. Whole-grain, cereal fiber, bran, and germ intake and the risks of all-cause and cardiovascular disease-specific mortality among women with type 2 diabetes mellitus. *Circulation* 2010;121:2162–2168

58. Thomas D, Elliott EJ. Low glycaemic index, or low glycaemic load, diets for diabetes mellitus. *Cochrane Database Syst Rev* 2009:CD006296

59. Westman EC, Yancy WS Jr, Mavropoulos JC, et al. The effect of a low-carbohydrate, ketogenic diet versus a low-glycemic index diet on glycemic control in type 2 diabetes mellitus. *Nutr Metab* 2008;5:36

60. Boeing H, Bechthold A, Bub A, et al. Critical review: vegetables and fruit in the prevention of chronic diseases. *Eur J Nutr* 2012;51:637–663

61. Elwood PC, Pickering JE, Givens DI, Gallacher JE. The consumption of milk and dairy foods and the incidence of vascular disease and diabetes: an overview of the evidence. *Lipids* 2010;45:925–939

62. Malik VS, Popkin BM, Bray GA, et al. Sugar-sweetened beverages and risk of metabolic syndrome and type 2 diabetes: a meta-analysis. *Diabetes Care* 2010;33:2477–2483

63. Hu FB, Malik VS. Sugar-sweetened beverages and risk of obesity and type 2 diabetes: epidemiologic evidence. *Physiol Behav* 2010;100:47–54

64. Imamura F, O'Connor L, Ye Z, et al. Consumption of sugar sweetened beverages, artificially sweetened beverages, and fruit juice and incidence of type 2 diabetes: systematic review, meta-analysis, and estimation of population attributable fraction. *BMJ* 2015;351:h3576

65. Peters AL, Davidson MB, Eisenberg K. Effect of isocaloric substitution of chocolate cake for potato in type I diabetic patients. *Diabetes Care* 1990;13:888–892

66. Fernandez ML, West KL. Mechanisms by which dietary fatty acids modulate plasma lipids. *J Nutr* 2005;135:2075–2078

67. Brunerova L, Smejkalova V, Potockova J, Andel M. A comparison of the influence of a high-fat diet enriched in monounsaturated fatty acids and conventional diet on weight loss and metabolic parameters in obese nondiabetic and type 2 diabetic patients. *Diabet Med* 2007;24:533–540

68. Weitz D, Weintraub H, Fisher E, Schwartzbard AZ. Fish oil for the treatment of cardiovascular disease. *Cardiol Rev* 2010;18:258–263

69. Bosch J, Gerstein HC, Dagenais GR, et al. n-3 Fatty acids and cardiovascular outcomes in patients with dysglycemia. *N Engl J Med* 2012;367:309–318

70. Gannon MC, Nuttall FQ, Saeed A, Jordan K, Hoover H. An increase in dietary protein improves the blood glucose response in persons with type 2 diabetes. *Am J Clin Nutr* 2003;78:734–741

71. Layman DK, Clifton P, Gannon MC, Krauss RM, Nuttall FQ. Protein in optimal health: heart disease and type 2 diabetes. *Am J Clin Nutr* 2008;87:1571S–1575S

72. Robertson L, Waugh N, Robertson A. Protein restriction for diabetic renal disease. *Cochrane Database Syst Rev* 2007:CD002181

73. Pan Y, Guo LL, Jin HM. Low-protein diet for diabetic nephropathy: a meta-analysis of randomized controlled trials. *Am J Clin Nutr* 2008;88:660–666

74. Teixeira SR, Tappenden KA, Carson L, et al. Isolated soy protein consumption reduces urinary albumin excretion and improves the serum lipid profile in men with type 2 diabetes mellitus and nephropathy. *J Nutr* 2004;134:1874–1880

75. Azadbakht L, Atabak S, Esmaillzadeh A. Soy protein intake, cardiorenal indices, and C-reactive protein in type 2 diabetes with nephropathy: a longitudinal randomized clinical trial. *Diabetes Care* 2008;31:648–654

76. Jayagopal V, Albertazzi P, Kilpatrick ES, et al. Beneficial effects of soy phytoestrogen intake in postmenopausal women with type 2 diabetes. *Diabetes Care* 2002;25:1709–1714

77. Bray GA, Vollmer WM, Sacks FM, et al. A further subgroup analysis of the effects of the DASH diet and three dietary sodium levels on blood pressure: results of the DASH-Sodium Trial. *Am J Cardiol* 2004;94:222–227

78. Ekinci EI, Clarke S, Thomas MC, et al. Dietary salt intake and mortality in patients with type 2 diabetes. *Diabetes Care* 2011;34:703–709

79. Thomas MC, Moran J, Forsblom C, et al. The association between dietary sodium intake, ESRD, and all-cause mortality in patients with type 1 diabetes. *Diabetes Care* 2011;34:861–866

80. Maillot M, Drewnowski A. A conflict between nutritionally adequate diets and meeting the 2010 dietary guidelines for sodium. *Am J Prev Med* 2012;42:174–179

81. Evert AB, Boucher JL, Cypress M, et al. Nutrition therapy recommendations for the management of adults with diabetes. *Diabetes Care* 2014;37(Suppl. 1):S120–S143

82. Howard AA, Arnsten JH, Gourevitch MN. Effect of alcohol consumption on diabetes mellitus: a systematic review. *Ann Intern Med* 2004;140:211–219

83. Richardson T, Weiss M, Thomas P, Kerr D. Day after the night before: influence of evening alcohol on risk of hypoglycemia in patients with type 1 diabetes. *Diabetes Care* 2005;28:1801–1802

84. Burge MR, Zeise TM, Sobhy TA, et al. Low-dose ethanol predisposes elderly fasted patients with type 2 diabetes to sulfonylurea-induced low blood glucose. *Diabetes Care* 1999;22:2037–2043

85. Jakicic JM, Marcus BH, Lang W, Janney C. Effect of exercise on 24-month weight loss maintenance in overweight women. *Arch Intern Med* 2008;168:1550–1559

86. Blair SN. Evidence for success of exercise in weight loss and control. *Ann Intern Med* 1993;119:702–706

87. Catenacci VA, Wyatt HR. The role of physical activity in producing and maintaining weight loss. *Nat Clin Pract Endocrinol Metab* 2007;3:518–529

88. Colberg SR, Sigal RJ, Fernhall B, et al. Exercise and type 2 diabetes: the American College of Sports Medicine and the American Diabetes Association: joint position statement. *Diabetes Care* 2010;33:e147–167

89. U.S. Department of Health and Human Services, Public Health Service, Centers for Disease Control and Prevention, National Center for Chronic Disease Prevention and Health Promotion, Division of Nutrition and Physical Activity. General physical activities defined by level of intensity. 1999. Available at http://www.cdc.gov/nccdphp/dnpa/physical/pdf/PA_Intensity_table_2_1.pdf. Accessed December 2015

90. Boule NG, Kenny GP, Haddad E, Wells GA, Sigal RJ. Meta-analysis of the effect of structured exercise training on cardiorespiratory fitness in type 2 diabetes mellitus. *Diabetologia* 2003;46:1071–1081

91. Katzmarzyk PT, Church TS, Craig CL, Bouchard C. Sitting time and mortality from all causes, cardiovascular disease, and cancer. *Med Sci Sports Exerc* 2009;41:998–1005

92. Church TS, Blair SN, Cocreham S, et al. Effects of aerobic and resistance training on hemoglobin A1c levels in patients with type 2 diabetes: a randomized controlled trial. *JAMA* 2010;304:2253–2262

93. Sigal RJ, Kenny GP, Boule NG, et al. Effects of aerobic training, resistance training, or both on glycemic control in type 2 diabetes: a randomized trial. *Ann Intern Med* 2007;147:357–369

94. Cooper DM, Barstow TJ, Bergner A, Lee WN. Blood glucose turnover during high- and low-intensity exercise. *Am J Physiol* 1989;257:E405–E412

95. Nield L, Moore HJ, Hooper L, et al. Dietary advice for treatment of type 2 diabetes mellitus in adults. *Cochrane Database Syst Rev* 2007:CD004097

96. Boule NG, Haddad E, Kenny GP, et al. Effects of exercise on glycemic control and body mass in type 2 diabetes mellitus: a meta-analysis of controlled clinical trials. *JAMA* 2001;286:1218–1227

97. Sukala WR, Page R, Cheema BS. Exercise training in high-risk ethnic populations with type 2 diabetes: a systematic review of clinical trials. *Diabetes Res Clin Pract* 2012;97:206–216

98. Paffenbarger RS Jr, Hyde RT, Wing AL, Hsieh CC. Physical activity, all-cause mortality, and longevity of college alumni. *N Engl J Med* 1986;314:605–613

99. Blair SN, Kohl HW 3rd, Paffenbarger RS Jr, et al. Physical fitness and all-cause mortality: a prospective study of healthy men and women. *JAMA* 1989;262:2395–2401

100. Kokkinos P, Myers J, Nylen E, et al. Exercise capacity and all-cause mortality in African American and Caucasian men with type 2 diabetes. *Diabetes Care* 2009;32:623–628

101. Larsen JJ, Dela F, Madsbad S, et al. Interaction of sulfonylureas and exercise on glucose homeostasis in type 2 diabetic patients. *Diabetes Care* 1999;22:1647–1654

102. Chu L, Hamilton J, Riddell MC. Clinical management of the physically active patient with type 1 diabetes. *Phys Sportsmed* 2011;39:64–77

103. Marliss EB, Vranic M. Intense exercise has unique effects on both insulin release and its roles in glucoregulation: implications for diabetes. *Diabetes* 2002;51(Suppl. 1):S271–S283

104. Pop-Busui R, Evans GW, Gerstein HC, et al. Effects of cardiac autonomic dysfunction on mortality risk in the Action to Control Cardiovascular Risk in Diabetes (ACCORD) trial. *Diabetes Care* 2010;33:1578–1584

105. Spallone V, Ziegler D, Freeman R, et al. Cardiovascular autonomic neuropathy in diabetes: clinical impact, assessment, diagnosis, and management. *Diabetes Metab Res Rev* 2011;27:639–653

106. Balducci S, Iacobellis G, Parisi L, et al. Exercise training can modify the natural history of diabetic peripheral neuropathy. *J Diabetes Complications* 2006;20:216–223

Chapter 3
Glycemia

As discussed in Chapter 1, there is no longer any doubt that an A1C level <7.0% will delay, and possibly prevent, the microvascular (retinopathy and nephropathy) and neuropathic complications of diabetes in both type 1 and type 2 diabetes patients, especially if the A1C level has been maintained at <7.0% since early in the duration of the disease (Figure 1.1). The American Diabetes Association (ADA) suggests the following goals for glycemic control in most patients: preprandial glucose, 80–130 mg/dL; postprandial glucose, <180 mg/dL; A1C level, <7.0%. A1C value is referenced to a nondiabetic range of 4.0–6.0% in an assay standardized to the Diabetes Control and Complications Trial–based method. A value of 6.0% reflects an average glucose concentration of 125 mg/dL with an approximately 30 mg/dL increase for every 1% increase in the A1C level throughout the day and night.[1]

In some patients, a less stringent A1C goal may be more appropriate. These patients would include individuals with: 1) a history of severe hypoglycemia; 2) short life expectancy; 3) advanced diabetic complications, especially the microvascular ones, since A1C levels <7.0% at that point will not reverse these complications; 4) social and educational issues; 5) cognitive dysfunction; 6) psychiatric issues; and 7) drug access/cost issues. In these situations, we use an A1C goal of <8.0%.

PRINCIPLES OF TREATMENT

Patients with type 1 diabetes require insulin. Type 2 diabetes is a progressive disease. β-Cell function, which is decreased by about 50% at diagnosis, continues to decrease regardless of which therapies are used (Figure 3.1).[2] (Note that despite the widely held misconception that sulfonylurea [SU] agents exhaust β-cells more than other drugs, after an initial increase in insulin secretion, the decline of β-cell function, i.e., slope of the curve, is similar in patients treated by diet alone and metformin.) To date, no other noninsulin therapies have been shown to preserve insulin secretion. Therefore, although initial treatment with metformin (along with diet and exercise) is often successful, over time, more than one noninsulin drug is required. Eventually, insulin is necessary in the majority of patients with type 2 diabetes.

DOI: 10.2337/9781580406017.01 **45**

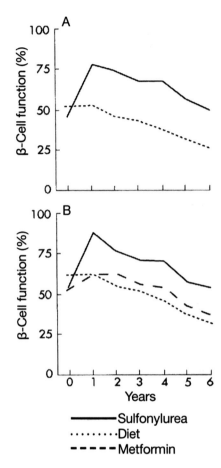

Figure 3.1. β-Cell function, as assessed by homoeostasis model assessment for patients in the UKPDS: (*A*) Subset of patients remaining on their allocated therapy at 6 years, comparing those allocated to diet (*n* = 376) and those allocated to sulfonylurea treatment (*n* = 511). (*B*) Subset of patients allocated to diet (*n* = 110) and those allocated to metformin (*n* = 159). Reprinted with permission from Holman.[2]

The 12 classes of drugs currently available to treat diabetes, along with their characteristics, are listed in Table 3.1.

Although all of these medications will be described, the following are the main drugs used in the U.S. and will be the focus of the remainder of this chapter: metformin, SUs, thiazolidinediones (TZDs), dipeptidyl peptidase (DPP)-4 inhibitors, glucagon-like peptide (GLP)-1 agonists, the sodium glucose transporter (SGLT)-2 inhibitors, and insulin. The α-glucosidase inhibitors are often used in other countries (e.g., China and Germany), but are not used frequently in this country because of their side effect of flatulence.

There are four criteria to use when selecting a class of drugs or a drug within a class from among its competitors: *1*) effectiveness; *2*) side effects; *3*) ease of use, which affects adherence to treatment; and *4*) cost/formulary availability. If the pro-

Table 3.1. Properties of available glucose-lowering agents in the U.S. that may guide individualized treatment choices in patients with type 2 diabetes.[3]

Class	Compound(s)	Cellular mechanism(s)	Primary physiological action(s)	Advantages	Disadvantages	Cost*
Biguanides	• Metformin	Activates AMP-kinase (? other)	• ↓ Hepatic glucose production	• Extensive experience • Rare hypoglycemia • ↓ ASCVD events (UKPDS) • Relatively higher A1C efficacy	• Gastrointestinal side effects (diarrhea, abdominal cramping, nausea) • Vitamin B12 deficiency • Contraindications: eGFR <30 mL/min/1.73 m², acidosis, hypoxia, dehydration, etc. • Lactic acidosis risk (rare)	Low
Sulfonylureas	2nd generation • Glyburide • Glipizide • Glimepiride	Closes K_{ATP} channels on β-cell plasma membranes	• ↑ Insulin secretion	• Extensive experience • ↓ Microvascular risk (UKPDS) • Relatively higher A1C efficacy	• Hypoglycemia • ↑ Weight	Low
Meglitinides (glinides)	• Repaglinide • Nateglinide	Closes K_{ATP} channels on β-cell plasma membranes	• ↑ Insulin secretion	• ↓ Postprandial glucose excursions • Dosing flexibility	• Hypoglycemia • ↑ Weight • Frequent dosing schedule	Moderate
TZDs	• Pioglitazone‡ • Rosiglitazone§	Activates the nuclear transcription factor PPAR-γ	• ↑ Insulin sensitivity	• Rare hypoglycemia • Relatively higher A1C efficacy • Durability • ↑ HDL cholesterol • ↓ Triglycerides (pioglitazone) • ? ↓ ASCVD events (PROactive, pioglitazone) • ↓ Risk of stroke and MI in patients without diabetes and with *insulin resistance* and history of recent stroke or TIA (IRIS study, pioglitazone)	• ↑ Weight • Edema/heart failure • Bone fractures • ↑ LDL cholesterol (rosiglitazone)	Low

(continued on page 48)

Table 3.1. Properties of available glucose-lowering agents in the U.S. that may guide individualized treatment choices in patients with type 2 diabetes.[3] (continued)

Class	Compound(s)	Cellular mechanism(s)	Primary physiological action(s)	Advantages	Disadvantages	Cost*
α-Glucosidase inhibitors	• Acarbose • Miglitol	Inhibits intestinal α-glucosidase	• Slows intestinal carbohydrate digestion/absorption	• Rare hypoglycemia • ↓ Postprandial glucose excursions • ? ↓ ASCVD events in prediabetes (STOP-NIDDM) • Nonsystemic	• Generally modest A1C efficacy • Gastrointestinal side effects (flatulence, diarrhea) • Frequent dosing schedule	Low to moderate
DPP-4 inhibitors	• Sitagliptin • Saxagliptin • Linagliptin • Alogliptin	Inhibits DPP-4 activity, increasing postprandial incretin (GLP-1, GIP) concentrations	• ↑ Insulin secretion (glucose dependent) • ↓ Glucagon secretion (glucose dependent)	• Rare hypoglycemia • Well tolerated	• Angioedema/urticaria and other immune-mediated dermatological effects • ? Acute pancreatitis • ↑ Heart failure hospitalizations (saxagliptin; ? alogliptin)	High
Bile acid sequestrants	• Colesevelam	Binds bile acids in intestinal tract, increasing hepatic bile acid production	• ? ↓ Hepatic glucose production • ? ↑ Incretin levels	• Rare hypoglycemia • ↓ LDL cholesterol	• Modest A1C efficacy • Constipation • ↑ Triglycerides • May ↓ absorption of other medications	High
Dopamine-2 agonists	• Bromocriptine (quick release)§	Activates dopaminergic receptors	• Modulates hypothalamic regulation of metabolism • ↑ Insulin sensitivity	• Rare hypoglycemia • ? ↓ ASCVD events (Cycloset Safety Trial)	• Modest A1C efficacy • Dizziness/syncope • Nausea • Fatigue • Rhinitis	High
SGLT2 inhibitors	• Canagliflozin • Dapagliflozin‡ • Empagliflozin	Inhibits SGLT2 in the proximal nephron	• Blocks glucose reabsorption by the kidney, increasing glucosuria	• Rare hypoglycemia • ↓ Weight • ↓ Blood pressure • Associated with lower ASCVD event rate and mortality in patients with ASCVD (empagliflozin EMPA-REG OUTCOME)	• Genitourinary infections • Polyuria • Volume depletion/hypotension/dizziness • ↑ LDL cholesterol • ↑ Creatinine (transient) • DKA, urinary tract infections leading to urosepsis, pyelonephritis	High

Class	Compound(s)	Cellular mechanism(s)	Physiological action(s)	Advantages	Disadvantages	Cost
GLP-1 receptor agonists	• Exenatide • Exenatide extended release • Liraglutide • Albiglutide • Lixisenatide • Dulaglutide	Activates GLP-1 receptors	• ↑ Insulin secretion (glucose dependent) • ↓ Glucagon secretion (glucose dependent) • Slows gastric emptying • ↑ Satiety	• Rare hypoglycemia • ↓ Weight • ↓ Postprandial glucose excursions • ↓ Some cardiovascular risk factors • Associated with lower ASCVD event rate and mortality in patients with ASCVD (liraglutide LEADER)	• Gastrointestinal side effects (nausea/vomiting/diarrhea) • ↑ Heart rate • ? Acute pancreatitis • C-cell hyperplasia/medullary thyroid tumors in animals • Injectable • Training requirements	High
Amylin mimetics	• Pramlintide§	Activates amylin receptors	• ↓ Glucagon secretion • Slows gastric emptying • ↑ Satiety	• ↓ Postprandial glucose excursions • ↓ Weight	• Modest A1C efficacy • Gastrointestinal side effects (nausea/vomiting) • Hypoglycemia unless insulin dose is simultaneously reduced • Injectable • Frequent dosing schedule • Training requirements	High

Insulins	• Rapid-acting analogs
	  – Lispro
	  – Aspart
	  – Glulisine
	  – Inhaled insulin
	• Short-acting
	  – Human Regular
	• Intermediate-acting
	  – Human NPH
	• Basal insulin analogs
	  – Glargine
	  – Detemir
	  – Degludec
	• Premixed insulin products
	  – NPH/Regular 70/30
	  – 70/30 aspart mix
	  – 75/25 lispro mix
	  – 50/50 lispro mix
		Activates insulin receptors	• ↑ Glucose disposal
			• ↓ Hepatic glucose production
			• Suppresses ketogenesis
				• Nearly universal response
				• Theoretically unlimited efficacy
				• ↓ Microvascular risk (UKPDS)
					• Hypoglycemia
					• Weight gain
					• Training requirements
					• Patient and provider reluctance
					• Injectable (except inhaled insulin)
					• Pulmonary toxicity (inhaled insulin)
						High#

ASCVD, atherosclerotic cardiovascular disease; EMPA-REG OUTCOME, BI 10773 (Empagliflozin) Cardiovascular Outcome Event Trial in Type 2 Diabetes Mellitus Patients[64]; GIP, glucose-dependent insulinotropic peptide; IRIS, Insulin Resistance Intervention After Stroke Trial[115]; LEADER, Liraglutide Effect and Action in Diabetes: Evaluation of Cardiovascular Outcome Results; PPAR-γ, peroxisome proliferator–activated receptor γ; PROactive, Prospective Pioglitazone Clinical Trial in Macrovascular Events[42]; STOP-NIDDM, Study to Prevent Non–Insulin–Dependent Diabetes Mellitus[116]; TIA, transient ischemic attack; TZD, thiazolidinedione; UKPDS, UK Prospective Diabetes Study.[117,118] Cycloset trial of quick-release bromocriptine.[67] *Cost is based on lowest-priced member of the class.[3] ‡Initial concerns regarding bladder cancer risk are decreasing after subsequent study. §Not licensed in Europe for type 2 diabetes. #Cost is highly dependent on type/brand (analogs > human insulins) and dosage. Adapted with permission from Inzucchi et al.[3]

vider feels that more than one choice would be appropriate, the pros and cons of each appropriate drug should be discussed with patients and their preferences should be taken into account.

Regarding effectiveness, A1C levels are used to judge the glycemic effect of drugs. It is important to realize that the higher the initial A1C level, the greater the fall after an intervention. Thus, when the older drugs (SUs and metformin) were tested earlier, glycemic control was generally worse than more recently when newer drugs were evaluated. This result would make the older drugs seem more effective because the decreases in A1C levels were greater. However, when compared with the newer drugs at comparable A1C levels, this result is not the case. Thus, when SUs, DPP-4 inhibitors, glinides, GLP-1 agonists, and α-glucosidase inhibitors or a placebo[4] are added to metformin[5] or to metformin plus an SU,[6] the A1C decreases were similar among the tested drugs. When these drugs were compared head-to-head,[7] the decreases were mostly similar (although in several studies, metformin was more effective than a DPP-4 inhibitor, and in one study, a TZD added to maximal doses of metformin plus an SU was more effective than an added DPP-4 inhibitor).[8] In head-to-head trials, the recently approved SGLT-2 inhibitors were also equally effective compared with metformin,[9] SUs,[10–12] and DPP-4 inhibitors.[9,13–17]

Although lifestyle modification (diet and exercise) should be used initially and reinforced throughout therapy, metformin should be started at diagnosis for the following reasons: *1*) even if diet and exercise alone may be effective initially, this regimen is difficult to sustain, and the vast majority of patients will soon require drug treatment; *2*) in the UK Prospective Diabetes Study (UKPDS), metformin was associated with less atherosclerotic cardiovascular disease (ASCVD) (at least two-thirds of patients with type 2 diabetes die from ASCVD); *3*) serious side effects to metformin are very rare; and *4*) metformin causes mild weight loss or at least weight stabilization.

Because no drug or class of drugs stands out as much more effective than any others (with the exception of insulin, which is the most effective if used appropriately), the other considerations for selecting treatments described previously take precedence. The ADA and the European Association for the Study of Diabetes (EASD) developed a Position Statement regarding the treatment of type 2 diabetes (Figure 3.2).[18]

We have adjusted their recommendations somewhat (Figure 3.3) based on our philosophy that as long as targets can be reached, the simpler the approach, the better for the patient (and in the case of insulin, for the provider as well). Because the mechanism of action of both SUs and DPP-4 inhibitors is to stimulate insulin secretion, we prefer to add another drug that has a different mechanism of action (although the DPP-4 inhibitors also decrease glucagon secretion). Therefore, if there are contraindications to a TZD and neither a GLP-1 agonist nor a SGLT-2 inhibitor is available, adding a DPP-4 inhibitor to an SU (or vice versa) could be considered.

Metformin, for which the major action is to reduce hepatic insulin resistance, is generally accepted as initial therapy. Our second-line therapy, either an SU or a DPP-4 inhibitor, stimulates insulin secretion, while the remaining three classes of noninsulin medications each have different major mechanisms of action; TZDs reduce peripheral insulin resistance; GLP-1 agonists, in addition to stimulating insulin secretion, suppress glucagon secretion (as do the DPP-4 inhibitors), reduce satiety leading to weight loss, and flatten postprandial glucose rises by inhibiting

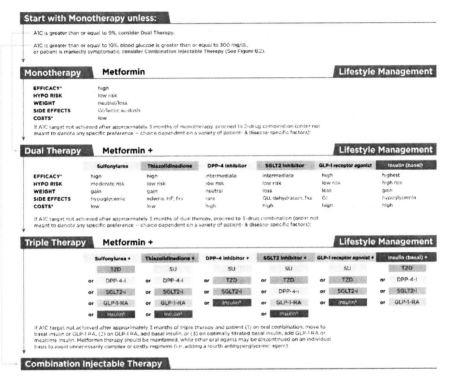

Figure 3.2. Antihyperglycemic therapy in type 2 diabetes: general recommendations. The order in the chart was determined by historical availability and the route of administration, with injectables to the right; it is not meant to denote any specific preference. Potential sequences of antihyperglycemic therapy for patients with type 2 diabetes are displayed, with the usual transition moving vertically from top to bottom (although horizontal movement within therapy stages is also possible, depending on the circumstances). DPP-4-i, DPP-4 inhibitor; fxs, fractures; GLP-1-RA, GLP-1 receptor agonist; GU, genitourinary; HF, heart failure; Hypo, hypoglycemia; SGLT2-i, SGLT2 inhibitor. *See Inzucchi et al.[3] for description of efficacy categorization. §Usually a basal insulin (NPH, glargine, detemir, degludec). Adapted with permission from Inzucchi et al.[3]

gastric emptying; and SGLT-2 inhibitors work by increasing glucosuria. Thus, each added class of medications should work synergistically by different mechanisms and be effective as long as insulin secretion is adequate enough (SGLT-2 inhibitors being the exception because they lower glycemia independent of insulin secretion).

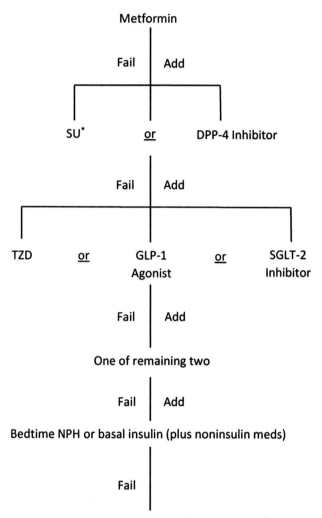

Figure 3.3. Flow diagram for treatment of patients with type 2 diabetes. See text for description of how to use each class of drugs. *Glinides may be substituted in patients with irregular eating patterns or in patients with late postpandrial hypoglycemia on an SU.

Regarding insulin therapy, we use it last in the progression of treatments for type 2 diabetes because it is an injection, requires self-monitoring of blood glucose (SMBG), has the potential for hypoglycemia, and can be associated with a less flexible lifestyle. Despite the recommendation to use it in severely hyperglycemic patients,[18] in newly diagnosed patients with type 2 diabetes, it is rarely necessary regardless of the initial glucose concentrations or A1C levels.[19–21] It is not clear why the ADA/EASD position statement gave only a passing mention to a less costly, two-injection, self-mixed/split insulin regimen with NPH and regular insulin. They recommend a premixed insulin regimen as an alternative to the basal/bolus regimen but admit that this two-injection regimen is inadequate to cover postprandial hyperglycemia, thus compromising achieving the A1C goal. We also do not use a combination of two drugs as initial therapy because it exposes the patient to more potential side effects and is more costly. Moreover, we quickly increase each drug to maximal doses so that after 3 months, we know whether more treatment is necessary. This step avoids having the patient who has achieved treatment goals continuing to take a drug that may not be necessary or avoids the hassle of either decreasing the dose or eliminating altogether one of the drugs used in the combination.

Two things must be stressed regarding the flow diagram in Figure 3.3. First, formulary issues may affect the suggested treatments. Second, and very importantly, when a therapy has failed, the patient must be advanced to the next therapy quickly. With some noninsulin drugs, failure is manifested by FPG concentrations above target several weeks after initiating or increasing the dose, while with others, it is an A1C level above target 3 months later (see below). The goal is to achieve an A1C level of <7.0% in most patients. However, there are five considerations to address before seeking this goal: *1*) limited life expectancy, *2*) the presence of advanced microvascular complications (tight control will have no effect at this point), *3*) severe ASCVD (tight control has little effect on ASCVD, and hypoglycemia can be detrimental), *4*) hypoglycemia unawareness (uncommon in patients with type 2 diabetes), and *5*) the inability or unwillingness to comply with the necessary regimen. In the absence of any of these, an A1C level of <7.0% should be sought.

USE OF NONINSULIN DRUGS

Patients with type 2 diabetes not taking insulin have a relatively stable FPG concentration.[22,23] A provider can take advantage of this when starting or titrating doses of metformin and an SU, two drugs that have a strong effect on fasting glycemia and show it within 2–3 weeks. This aspect of type 2 diabetes is not as helpful for drugs that have their major effects on postprandial glucose concentrations (α-glucosidase inhibitors, glinides, GLP-1 analogs, DPP-4 inhibitors, SGLT-2 inhibitors) or the TZDs with their delayed effect.

When a therapy has failed, the patient must be advanced to the next treatment promptly to achieve the glycemic targets quickly and avoid leaving the patient out of control for an extended period. The list of drugs used to treat type 2 diabetes and their cellular mechanisms, physiological actions, advantages, and disadvantages are shown in Table 3.1. Of course, formulary and cost issues will importantly influence the drugs available to an individual patient. As mentioned previously, if choices are possible, describing the pros and cons of each drug and eliciting the patient's input is helpful to maximize medication adherence.

METFORMIN (GLUCOPHAGE, GLUMETZA)

Principles of use

Because of the common (usually temporary) gastrointestinal (GI) adverse effects that occur when metformin is started or the dose is increased, it is important to start with a small dose (500 twice daily) and increase it gradually. If the patient experiences GI adverse effects, they will occur during the first week, usually with subsequent marked improvement or disappearance of these symptoms. (To minimize these symptoms, metformin should be taken with meals.) The FPG concentration should be measured 2–3 weeks after starting metformin and 2–3 weeks after each dose change. The FPG concentration can be measured in the laboratory, by a point-of-care glucose meter in the clinic or office, or, if the patient is considered reliable, by SMBG at home. In the latter case, we ask the patient to measure 3 consecutive days at the appropriate time interval after starting or increasing the dose. The short-term goal is to achieve a value of <130 mg/dL. If that goal is not achieved, and any GI symptoms that may be present are tolerable, the dose of metformin is increased by one step (see Table 3.2) until *1*) the FPG concentration becomes <130 mg/dL, *2*) the GI symptoms are intolerable (in

Table 3.2. Metformin Dosing Schedule

Total dose (mg)	Before breakfast	Before lunch	Before supper
500	500	—	—
1,000[a]	500	—	500
1,500	500	—	1,000[b]
2,000	1,000	—	1,000
OR			
850	850	—	—
1,700	850	—	850
2,550	850	850	850
OR			
Extended release			
500			500[c]
750[a]			750[c]
1,000[a]			1,000[c]
1,500			1,500[c]
2,000			2,000[c]
2,250			2,250[c]

Immediate-release forms are in 500-, 850-, and 1,000-mg tablets; extended-release forms are in 500-, 750-, and 1,000-mg tablets. [a]Usual starting dose. [b]Given with largest meal to minimize GI adverse events. [c]Given with supper or at bedtime.

which case, the dose should be reduced by one step), or *3*) the maximal dose is reached.

As long as the FPG concentration remains above 130 mg/dL, the dose of metformin should be increased by one step and the FPG concentration measured in 2–3 weeks until the value falls below 130 mg/dL, at which time the dose is maintained and FPG and A1C levels are measured 3 months later. If the A1C level is at the target level at that time (regardless of the FPG concentration), the dose of metformin is maintained, and both tests should be repeated every 3 months. On the other hand, if the A1C level is above the target level, the dose of metformin is increased by one step, or, if already at the maximal dose, an SU or a DPP-4 inhibitor is added. If an SU was added, the protocol for assessing a dose increase is then followed (i.e., measuring the FPG concentration in 2–3 weeks if it were ≥130 mg/dL). It is unnecessary to repeat the FPG concentration in 2–3 weeks if the target has been met (i.e., <130 mg/dL) and the dose increase or the addition of an SU occurred because the A1C was above target. In that case, the FPG and A1C levels should be repeated in 3 months and the evaluation process detailed here should be followed. If a DPP-4 inhibitor was added, see "DPP-4 Inhibitors" for dosing instructions.

Random plasma glucose versus FPG

Because it is inconvenient for most patients to obtain an FPG, either in the clinic or office or at a laboratory, and most of them are seen during the day, a random plasma glucose (RPG) can be used instead of an FPG to evaluate a patient's control. The RPG depends on two factors: the amount of carbohydrate in the preceding meal and the amount of elapsed time from that meal. The more carbohydrate ingested, the higher the postprandial glucose concentration with a maximum value usually reached between 1 and 2 hours after the meal. The ADA's postprandial glucose target is <180 mg/dL.[1] Because most patients will not be sampled 1–2 hours after eating, we use a RPG target of <160 mg/dL. Therefore, RPG concentrations exceeding this value can be used instead of an FPG concentration of <130 mg/dL to increase the dose of metformin or add another noninsulin drug if the patient is already taking the maximal (tolerated) dose of the biguanide. This step also applies to the titration of an SU.

Whenever intolerable GI symptoms to metformin occur, the dose should be reduced by one step and the patient reevaluated. This adverse effect will usually occur after a dose increase, which implies that satisfactory control had not yet been achieved before the increase. In this case, adding a second drug should be strongly considered. If, on the other hand, intolerable GI symptoms occur after the patient has been on a stable dose of metformin, an A1C level should be measured 3 months after the one-step decrease in dose. If the value is at target, the dose is maintained and the patient evaluated with A1C levels every 3 months. If the value is above target, either an SU or a DPP-4 inhibitor should be added.

If the maximal dose of metformin is reached and the patient is in unsatisfactory control (i.e., an FPG concentration ≥130 mg/dL 2–3 weeks after the final dose increase or an A1C level is above target 3 months after the last evaluation), either an SU or a DPP-4 inhibitor should be added.

Incremental step doses and maximal final doses

Metformin is marketed in tablets containing 500, 850, and 1,000 mg of the drug and in an extended-release form containing 500, 750, and 1,000 mg. The extended-release forms may have fewer GI adverse events. The original studies with the 500-mg tablets suggested that the maximal dose was 2,500 mg. A subsequent dose-response study revealed that there was no additional effect over 2,000 mg.[24] Therefore, if the 500-mg tablet is used, there are usually only three steps (the usual starting dose is 500 mg twice a day), and the patient should take the tablets only twice daily. If the 850-mg tablet is used, there are also only three steps, and the patient takes the tablets three times a day with each meal. If the 1,000-mg tablets are used, there are two steps: 1,000 mg once daily and 1,000 mg twice daily. The extended-release forms need to be taken only once daily and are recommended by the manufacturers to be ingested with the evening meal or at bedtime. The starting dose is either 750 or 1,000 mg, with only a one-step increase for the 1,000-mg tablet (or two 500-mg tablets) to a maximal dose of 2,000 mg or a two-step increase for the 750-mg tablet to a maximal dose of 2,250 mg. Table 3.2 describes the dosing schedule of various metformin tablet sizes.

Contraindications

Renal insufficiency (previously a serum creatinine >1.4 mg/dL for women and >1.5 mg/dL for men) was a contraindication, but that is no longer the case. Estimated glomerular filtration rates (eGFRs) are now used,[25] and recent evidence[26] indicates that metformin can safely be used down to eGFRs of 30 mL/min/1.73 m² (stage 3B kidney disease); however, if used in patients with stage 3B kidney disease (30–45 mL/min/1.73 m²), the maximal dose should be reduced to 1,000 mg/day.[18]

Other contraindications
- Hepatic dysfunction: alanine transaminase (ALT) or aspartate transaminase (AST) more than three times normal (metformin does not cause hepatic dysfunction; the concern is that impaired liver function will be unable to metabolize lactate, facilitating the potential of lactic acidosis; however, this is unlikely because the liver has a tremendous ability to metabolize lactate and lactic acidosis is probably not related to metformin [see below])
- History of alcoholism or binge drinking (since the metabolism of ethanol may lead to an accumulation of lactate)
- Acute or chronic metabolic acidosis

Discontinuation

The drug should be temporarily discontinued until the following circumstances are no longer present: *a*) acute myocardial infarction, *b*) major surgery, or *c*) severe infection. Recognizing that it is safe to use metformin down to an eGFR of 30 mL/min/1.73 m²,[26] in 2015, the American College of Radiology stopped recommending temporarily discontinuing metformin for imaging studies using intravenous contrast material (dye studies).[27]

Serious adverse events

Because phenformin, a biguanide like metformin, was pulled from the U.S. market for causing lactic acidosis, it has been assumed that this complication with its high mortality could also be caused by metformin. Although lactic acidosis can occur rarely in patients taking metformin (approximately four cases per 100,000 patients), the rate is no different than that occurring in diabetes patients taking other medications for diabetes[28] and is probably related to underlying morbidity rather than to metformin per se.[29] Furthermore, just about all cases occurring in patients exposed to metformin have occurred in patients in whom the drug was contraindicated, with the great majority having marked renal insufficiency.

SULFONYLUREA AGENTS AND GLINIDES

Principles of use: SUs

Since the first-generation SUs (acetoheximade, chlorpropamide, tolazamide, tolbutamide) are used so rarely, this discussion will be limited to the second-generation SUs and those available in this country (glimeperide, glipizide, and glyburide). Because of its greater propensity to cause hypoglycemia and no greater effectiveness than the other two second-generation SUs, glyburide is no longer recommended. The starting and maximal doses of the second-generation SUs are listed in Table 3.3. The FPG concentration should be measured 2–3 weeks after starting an SU and after each dose change. As with metformin, the short-term goal is to achieve a value of <130 mg/dL. If that goal is not achieved, the dose of the SU is increased in one-step increments (see "Incremental Step Doses" below) until either the goal is met or the maximal dose of the SU is reached. When an FPG concentration of <130 mg/dL is achieved, an A1C level and an FPG concentration should be measured 3 months later.

Table 3.3. Starting and Maximal Doses (mg) of the Second-Generation SUs and Glinides

Generic name	Brand name	Starting[a]	Maximal
Glyburide	Micronase	5	20
Glyburide	Glynase	3	12
Glipizide	Glucotrol	10	40
Glipizide	Glucotrol XL	5	20
Glimepiride	Amaryl	2	8
Repaglinide	Prandin	1[b]	Usually 12[c]
Nateglinide	Starlix	120[b]	360

[a]Lower starting doses are often recommended, but in our experience, higher doses are almost always needed. [b]Before each meal. [c]Maximum dose is 4 mg per meal (16 mg if a fourth meal is eaten, but a dose is usually not taken for a small bedtime snack); if a meal is missed, that dose (whatever the amount) should be omitted.

The long-term goal is to achieve the target A1C level in the absence of unexplained hypoglycemia (unexplained hypoglycemia is described under "Insulin" below). When this goal is achieved, A1C levels and FPG concentrations can be measured every 3 months. As mentioned previously, if measurements of FPG concentrations by the patient are considered reliable, the average of 3 days of consecutive values may be substituted for a laboratory-measured value. (All glucose meters are calibrated to give plasma levels.) Fingerstick blood samples reflect capillary glucose concentrations that are similar to the values measured in the laboratory from a venipuncture sample as long as the patient is in the fasting state. (Random and postprandial values are higher in capillary samples, the difference depending on how long ago the patient ate and the carbohydrate content of the meal.) Whenever FPG concentrations are mentioned in these protocols concerning noninsulin drugs, measurements of FPG concentrations on 3 consecutive days by reliable patients can be substituted for the laboratory-measured value.

If the maximal dose of the SU is reached (plus metformin unless contraindicated), and the FPG concentration 2–3 weeks later is ≥180 mg/dL or an A1C level 3 months later is greater than target, a noninsulin medication should be added if available for the patient and, of course, not contraindicated. If the FPG concentration 2–3 weeks after the maximal dose of the SU is reached is 130–179 mg/dL, the A1C level measured 3 months later drives the decision whether or not to add a third medication. Some patients taking an SU will have a moderately elevated FPG concentration but an A1C level at target, presumably because the SU via enhanced insulin secretion keeps the glucose levels reasonably low during the day, even though they start out >130 mg/dL. Diet and exercise should be stressed during this period, so that the patient can avoid adding the third medication. *All patients starting an SU or a glinide must be taught the signs, symptoms, and treatment of hypoglycemia.*

Principles of use: glinides

Repaglinide and nateglinide are drugs that like SUs also stimulate β-cells to secrete more insulin. They bind to a different part of the same receptor to which the SUs bind. The difference is that the β-cells respond more quickly to glinides and only for a short period of time, leading to rapid increases in insulin concentrations that quickly return to baseline levels. Therefore, there is somewhat less hypoglycemia in patients taking glinides compared with SUs. These drugs are advantageous for patients who have irregular eating patterns. A disadvantage is that they must be taken before each meal, usually three times a day. The starting and maximal doses of the glinides are listed in Table 3.3.

Incremental step doses

The dosing schedules for the SUs and glinides are shown in Table 3.4.

THIAZOLIDINEDIONES (GLITAZONES)

Mechanism of action

TZDs bind to a nuclear receptor (called the peroxisome proliferator–activated receptor-γ, or PPAR-γ). This binding results in activation of a gene or genes that

Table 3.4. Dosing Schedule[a] for Second-Generation SUs and Glinides

Total dose (mg)	Before breakfast	Before lunch	Before supper
Glyburide (Micronase, DiaBeta)			
(1.25)	(1.25)	—	—
(2.5)	(2.5)	—	—
5	5	—	—
10	10	—	—
15	10	—	5
20	10	—	10
Micronized glyburide (Glynase)			
(1.5)	(1.5)	—	—
3	3	—	—
6	6	—	—
9	6	—	3
12	6	—	6
Glipizide (Glucotrol)			
(2.5)	(2.5)		
(5)	(5)	—	—
10	5	—	5
20	10	—	10
40	20	—	20
Extended-release glipizide (Glucotrol XL)			
(2.5)	(2.5)	—	—
5	5	—	—
10	10	—	—
20	20	—	—
Glimepiride[b] (Amaryl)			
(1)	(1)	—	—
2	2	—	—
4	4	—	—
8	8	—	—
Repaglinide[c] (Prandin)			
(1.5)	(0.5)	(0.5)	(0.5)
3	1.0	1.0	1.0
6	2.0	2.0	2.0
12	4.0	4.0	4.0
Nateglinide (Starlix)			
360	120	120	120

[a]Manufacturers' recommended initial doses smaller than those used in the protocols are in parentheses. [b]May be taken at any time of the day. [c]Maximum dose is 16 mg if a fourth meal is eaten.

increase(s) glucose utilization (probably by increasing glucose transport) in muscle and fat tissue. In this manner, TZDs decrease peripheral insulin resistance, which is an important characteristic of type 2 diabetes. They also have a more minor effect on reducing hepatic insulin resistance leading to decreased hepatic glucose production.

Clinical use

The U.S. Food and Drug Administration (FDA) has approved two TZDs (rosiglitazone [Avandia] and pioglitazone [Actos]) for use in patients with type 2 diabetes. (These drugs are not indicated for patients with type 1 diabetes.) They can be used as monotherapy, in combination with other oral anti-hyperglycemic drugs, or with insulin. TZDs take 2–4 weeks before an effect can be seen (consistent with their mechanism of action affecting gene expression) with a maximal effect not evident for 3–4 months. Rosiglitazone is marketed in 2-, 4-, and 8-mg tablets. Pioglitazone is marketed in 15-, 30-, and 45-mg tablets. Because a maximum response to a glitazone may take up to 4 months, if a patient starts with a submaximal dose with a plan to increase it if an inadequate response is documented, it may take the better part of a year before knowing whether the patient will have an adequate response to the glitazone. For this reason, we start the patient with the maximum dose: 8 mg once a day for rosiglitazone and 45 mg once a day for pioglitazone. With this approach, it will take 4 months to know whether the patient will have an adequate response to the glitazone (see below for criteria for starting insulin). Because all of these patients will be on a maximal dose of an SU, measure the FPG concentration 2 months after starting the glitazone to ascertain that the patient is not hypoglycemic. If the FPG concentration is <70 mg/dL (or if the patient is having hypoglycemic episodes), the dose of the SU, *not the glitazone*, should be reduced.

Adverse effects

Troglitazone (Rezulin), the first approved TZD, was removed from the market because of rare, but sometimes fatal, hepatic failure. These episodes were preceded by elevations in hepatic transaminases, especially ALT. Although there were no differences in increases in ALT levels between patients receiving placebo and those receiving either rosiglitazone or pioglitazone during preapproval clinical studies, because of the structural similarity among the three TZDs, the FDA initially recommended that patients receiving the two newer ones also have their hepatic function monitored until more experience with them was obtained. Based on the post-marketing extensive experience with both rosiglitazone and pioglitazone and the lack of evidence of hepatic dysfunction attributed to these drugs, the FDA removed the requirement for ongoing liver function testing in the absence of another clinical reason for it. However, the FDA still recommends that ALT levels be measured before starting rosiglitazone or pioglitazone. Neither drug should be used if ALT levels are more than three times the upper limit of normal.

TZDs increase the plasma volume slightly by increasing fluid retention. This increased plasma volume results in a clinically insignificant lowering of the hematocrit and hemoglobin level and the white blood cell count, and the fluid retention may help account for some of the weight gain noted in some patients. The increase in fluid retention may also cause or worsen edema, as well as heart failure, in individuals who already have either condition or are prone to getting either one. These drugs were not studied in patients with New York Heart Association Class III or IV cardiac status and should be avoided in these individuals. Therefore, TZDs should be used with caution in patients with a history of edema. TZD use is not advised in patients who have edema already present or a history of heart failure.

If peripheral edema occurs, the dose of the glitazone can be reduced (halved to 4 mg once a day for rosiglitazone and decreased to 30 mg once a day for pioglitazone) or discontinued. Because we do not start a glitazone in patients with edema, few of our patients have developed edema, even on the maximal doses. If patients do develop edema that persists after the dose of the glitazone is reduced, we prefer to discontinue the drug rather than to add a diuretic. When glitazones are discontinued, another noninsulin drug should be substituted, if available. Keep in mind that just as the onset of action of glitazones is delayed, so is the waning of their effect. Therefore, although initially it may seem as if the substituted drug is maintaining the patient in satisfactory control, this may not be the case several months later.

Glitazones are associated with decreased bone mineral density[30] and increased fractures, although there is more of a risk in women.[31]

A 5-year interim report of a large 10-year study evaluating a possible association of pioglitazone with bladder cancer showed no significant association in the primary outcome, ever versus never use of the drug, but there was a significant association in a secondary outcome in patients who used the drug for more than 2 years.[32] However, the final 10-year report did not confirm these findings, with again no association comparing ever versus never use of the drug but also no association in patients who had used pioglitazone for more than 4 years.[33]

Furthermore, there are 14 other negative studies showing no association between bladder cancer and the use of pioglitazone.[34] Thus, the initial concern about a potential increased risk of bladder cancer in patients exposed to pioglitazone was not borne out, and in our view, is not a factor in the use of pioglitazone.

Lipid effects

TZDs have varying effects on lipids. Total cholesterol and LDL cholesterol concentrations are increased by both rosiglitazone and pioglitazone, but more so with rosiglitazone. HDL cholesterol concentrations are also increased by both glitazones, but more so with pioglitazone. Neither the total cholesterol/HDL cholesterol nor the LDL cholesterol/HDL cholesterol ratios changed appreciably in patients receiving rosiglitazone and pioglitazone. Moreover, the LDL particle shifted from a more atherogenic small dense particle size to a less atherogenic large fluffy one with both glitazones. Finally, fasting triglyceride concentrations were decreased by pioglitazone but not by rosiglitazone.

Miscellaneous

Dose adjustments of the two glitazones are not necessary in the elderly or in patients with renal insufficiency. Some anovulatory women with polycystic ovary syndrome (PCOS) have ovulated, and a few have conceived when receiving metformin alone. This result is presumably due to the reduction of insulin resistance, which characterizes PCOS, leading to a reduction of hyperandrogenism and improvement in gonadotropin secretion. Adding clomiphene increases the fertility rate considerably. Glitazones have been used to treat women with PCOS.[35] Because they cause intrauterine growth retardation in animal studies, glitazones should be discontinued immediately if conception occurs in women with PCOS. Appropriate contraception is advised for those women with PCOS receiving glitazones (or metformin) who do not wish to become pregnant.

Which glitazone?

In response to a meta-analysis based on data pooled from 42 small clinical trials that allegedly showed a 43% increase in myocardial infarctions in patients exposed to rosiglitazone,[36] the FDA severely restricted its use. Subsequent experience in 4,500 patients did not support that conclusion,[37] and the FDA recently lifted their restrictions allowing rosiglitazone to be freely used once more.[38] On the other hand, accumulating evidence strongly suggests that pioglitazone may actually have a direct beneficial effect on ASCVD and its events. In randomized control trials in patients with type 2 diabetes, pioglitazone had a significant beneficial effect on: *1)* the surrogate markers of ASCVD of carotid intima thickness[39] and intravascular coronary imaging by ultrasound[40]; *2)* restenosis after coronary artery stent placement[41]; *3)* the composite of mortality, myocardial infarction, and stroke[42,43]; *4)* recurrent myocardial infarctions and acute coronary syndrome[44]; *5)* recurrent strokes[45]; and *6)* peripheral arterial disease.[46,47] Pioglitazone is also preferred because of its more favorable effect on lipids, which may be related to its beneficial effects on ASCVD.

INCRETINS

Background

It was shown nearly 50 years ago that glucose given by mouth elicits a greater insulin response than amounts given intravenously at similar attained glucose concentrations. The difference in insulin levels between oral and intravenous administration (despite similar plasma glucose concentrations) is called the "incretin effect" and was postulated to involve factors secreted by the gastrointestinal tract after oral glucose ingestion. One of these factors is the hormone GLP-1. Within minutes after starting a meal, the L-cells in the distal ileum secrete GLP-1. Although food has obviously not reached the distal ileum at this time, K-cells in the upper duodenum signal the brain (via vagus pathways) to stimulate the L-cells to secrete GLP-1. The half-life of GLP-1 in the circulation is only 2 minutes because the enzyme DPP-4 quickly inactivates the hormone. Although GLP-1 and glucagon share some homology in their amino acid structures (hence the similarity of their names), their actions are much different. Glucagon is a counterregulatory hormone that increases hepatic glucose production. In contrast, GLP-1 inhibits glucagon secretion, stimulates insulin secretion in a glucose-dependent manner, slows gastric emptying, and suppresses appetite. The glucose-dependent aspect of stimulating insulin secretion means that the increase in insulin release only occurs when glucose concentrations are elevated, not when they are normal, and, therefore, incretins (by themselves) do not cause hypoglycemia.

Although a possible signal of pancreatitis associated with incretin use was detected by adverse event reports after FDA approval of the drugs, a review of observational studies in which confounders for pancreatitis were taken into account could find no significant association of pancreatitis with these drugs.[48] Similarly, a possible signal for pancreatic cancer was also suggested in adverse event reports[48] but could not be substantiated[49-51] in subsequent epidemiological studies.

Incretin analogs (GLP-1 agonists)

The saliva of the Gila monster (a large lizard) contains a compound that shares homology with GLP-1 but with a difference occurring at the site where DPP-4 inactivates GLP-1. Therefore, DPP-4 does not inactivate these compounds, allowing them half-lives of many hours after subcutaneous injection. By virtue of the ability of GLP-1 agonists to suppress glucagon (which is normally suppressed after eating, but not in people with diabetes), to stimulate insulin secretion, and to delay gastric emptying, the postprandial rise of glucose is blunted. Fasting glucose concentrations also decrease but not as much as postprandial concentrations. GLP-1 agonists also decrease appetite, resulting in weight loss in many patients, which in turn increases insulin sensitivity, also resulting in improved diabetes control. Several GLP-1 agonists have been marketed, and some have been fused to serum proteins or to a polymer, markedly extending their half-lives (Table 3.5).

Up to 30% of patients receiving GLP-1 agonists experience nausea that is usually mild and often gradually disappears over several weeks to a month. The weight loss is slightly greater in these patients but is also seen in patients without nausea. On average, weight loss (~10 lb) has been maintained for over 1 year. Because of the glucose dependence of insulin secretion, GLP-1 agonists by themselves do not cause hypoglycemia. However, because patients who are also receiving an SU may experience hypoglycemia, the dose of the SU (or glinide) should

Table 3.5. Marketed GLP-1 Agonists

Generic name	Brand name	Mixing required	Pre-injection waiting time	Dosing schedule	Doses
Exenatide	Byetta	No	None	Twice per day	5 and 10 µg
Liraglutide	Victoza	No	None	Once per day	0.6, 1.2, and 1.8 mg
Lixisenatide	Adlyxin	No	None	Once per day	10 and 20 µg
Exenatide extended release	Bydureon	Yes	None	Once per week	2 mg
Trulicity	Dulaglutide	No	None	Once per week	0.75 and 1.5 mg
Tanzeum	Albiglutide	Yes	15–30 minutes	Once per week	30 and 50 mg

be halved when a GLP-1 agonist is started. If hypoglycemia does not occur, the SU dose should be maximized again.

Clinical use. In keeping with the principle of maximizing the dose of a medication (if not curtailed by side effects) to ascertain quickly whether the target has been achieved or a drug from another class is necessary (thereby minimizing the time a patient remains uncontrolled), we rapidly increase the dose of those GLP-1 agonists with two recommended doses. The initial dose of exenatide is 5 µg twice daily for the first month, increasing to 10 µg twice daily, the maximal approved dose, if side effects allow after the first month. The 0.6 mg dose of liraglutide is given for only 1 week to minimize the GI side effects as higher doses are used; this lower dose does not have much of a glycemic effect. The dose is increased to 1.2 mg for the next 3 weeks, and then if side effects allow, to 1.8 mg. The initial dose of lixisenatide is 10 µg per day for 2 weeks followed by an increase to 20 µg per day. The lower doses of dulaglutide and albiglutide are used for 1 month and increased to the higher doses at that time, again if side effects allow. Three months after the GLP-1 agonists are started, an A1C level should be measured to determine if the target level has been achieved. If so, they are continued with A1C levels every 3 months to decide if they should be continued (target level maintained) or if another class of drugs should be introduced (target level exceeded).

Other effects. Two GLP-1 agonists, liraglutide in the LEADER (Liraglutide Effect and Action in Diabetes: Evaluation of Cardiovascular Outcome Results) trial[52] and semaglutide (not yet approved) in the SUSTAIN-6 (Trial to Evaluate Cardiovascular and Other Long-term Outcomes with Semaglutide in Subjects with Type 2 Diabetes) trial,[53] had significantly beneficial effects on ASCVD; however, a third GLP-1 agonist, lixisenatide in the ELIXA (Evaluation of Lixisenatide in Acute Coronary Syndrome) trial, did not.[54]

DPP-4 inhibitors

Compounds that inhibit the DPP-4 enzyme should allow endogenous GLP-1 to remain active for longer periods of time. A single oral dose of a DPP-4 inhibitor maintains its inhibition of the enzyme for >24 h and thereby increases the postprandial response of GLP-1 for >24 h. As with the GLP-1 agonists, FPG concentrations are decreased somewhat but not nearly as much as postprandial concentrations. The maximal lowering of FPG concentrations occurs by 1 month with no further decline. DPP-4 inhibitors have a benign side effect profile.[55] Unlike GLP-1 agonists, they are weight-neutral. Because GLP-1 stimulates insulin secretion in a glucose-dependent manner, DPP-4 inhibitors also do not cause hypoglycemia. Increased hospitalizations for heart failure were reported in patients using saxagliptin,[56] but this result was not confirmed for saxagliptin or the other DPP-4 inhibitors in two studies that used two large administrative databases.[57,58]

Clinical use. DPP-4 inhibitors are taken once per day (with one exception), but their dose may be affected by renal function, as described in Table 3.6.

There are two possible ways to follow patients prescribed a DPP-4 inhibitor. The easiest is to simply wait 3 months and measure an A1C level. If the level is at target, continue the medication, measuring A1C levels every 3 months. If the A1C level is above target, add a medication from one of the three recommended classes

Table 3.6. Effect of Renal Function on Doses of DPP-4 Inhibitors

DPP-4 inhibitor	eGFR (mL/min)	Dose (mg q.d. unless noted otherwise)
Alogliptin (Nesina)	≥60 ≥30 to <60 <30	25 12.5 6.25
Linagliptin (Tradjenta)	Any	5
Saxagliptin (Onglyza)	>50 ≤50	5 2.5
Sitagliptin (Januvia)	≥50 ≥30 to <50 <30	100 50 25
Vildagliptin (Galvus)	≥60 <60	50 mg (b.i.d.) 50 mg

of drugs (Figure 3.3). The other way to monitor is to follow the principle of determining quickly whether the current treatment will achieve target. The tactic differs from following patients who start a GLP-1 agonist because even if their glycemic response at 1 month is not satisfactory, their continued weight loss may improve control after that time. In contrast, because DPP-4 inhibitors are weight neutral, weight loss is not a factor in their glycemic effect. Because incretins improve postprandial glycemia more than fasting glycemia, we use an FPG concentration 1 month after starting a DPP-4 inhibitor of 150 mg/dL or a RPG of 180 mg/dL (rather than of 130 mg/dL and 160 mg/dL, respectively, for metformin and SUs) to decide whether to add another therapy. If the FPG value is <150 mg/dL or the RPG value is <180 mg/dL, the DPP-4 inhibitor is continued and the A1C level in 2 more months determines the next step. If the FPG or RPG values are ≥150 or 180 mg/dL, respectively, a drug from one of the recommended classes of drugs is added (Figure 3.3).

SGLT-2 INHIBITORS

Although all of the glucose in the circulation is filtered at the renal glomeruli and flows through the kidney, in people without diabetes, none appears in the urine. This absence of glucosuria occurs because all of the glucose is reabsorbed back into the circulation, 90% by activity of the enzyme SGLT-2 located in the initial segment of the proximal convoluted renal tubule and the remaining 10% by SGLT-1 located further down the proximal segment. The reabsorption of filtered glucose increases linearly until the maximal reabsorptive capacity (T_m) is exceeded, at which point glucose begins to appear in the urine. The plasma glucose concentration at which this normally occurs in adults is approximately 180 mg/dL and is referred to as the renal threshold. The renal threshold increases with age and is markedly lower in pregnancy. Inhibitors of SGLT-2 result in marked glucosuria, which lowers plasma glucose concentrations. A major advantage of SGLT-2 inhibitors is that they do not require insulin secretion for their effect, a process that progressively diminishes as the duration of type 2 diabetes increases (Figure 3.1). Renal function affects the use of the SGLT-2 inhibitors (Table 3.7).

Adverse effects

Patients taking an SGLT-2 inhibitor obviously experience polyuria and some nocturia. This increased urination can cause dehydration unless patients ingest enough fluids to counterbalance the fluid loss. Additionally, urinary tract infections (6.3% vs. 4.7%) and genital mycotic infections (6.5% vs. 1.3%) are more common in patients taking SGLT-2 inhibitors compared with placebos or another comparator.[59] These infections are more likely to occur in women than in men. Because balanitis is more common in the uncircumcized male, instruction in penile hygiene is helpful to reduce this risk. Diabetic ketoacidosis (DKA) has been rarely reported in <0.1% of patients with type 2 diabetes taking an SGLT-2 inhibitor,[60] although it is noted much more commonly (~5%) in patients with type 1 diabetes exposed to the drugs off label.[61] Glucose concentrations can be <250 mg/dL at the time of diagnosis in DKA associated with SGLT-2 inhibitors. The FDA has recently updated its warnings on DKA and severe urosepsis.[62] Finally, there is a suggestion that SGLT-2 inhibitors may be associated with an increased risk of fractures.[63]

Other effects

There is a mild weight loss of 2.2 kg and a slight lowering of systolic blood pressure of 3.7 mmHg in patients taking SGLT-2 inhibitors.[58] One SGLT-2 inhibitor (empagliflozin) had a beneficial effect on ASCVD events, death from ASCVD, and hospitalizations for heart failure.[64] This result may be a class effect; studies with other SGLT-2 inhibitors are ongoing.

Clinical use

SGLT-2 inhibitors are taken once a day. We start with the lowest dose. As with GLP-1 agonists, in keeping with the principle of maximizing the dose of a medication (if not curtailed by adverse effects, or in this case, by the eGFR) to ascertain quickly whether the target has been achieved or a drug from another class is necessary (thereby minimizing the time a patient remains uncontrolled), we increase the dose of the SGLT-2 inhibitor to the maximal dose where possible after 1 month. An A1C level 2 months later (3 months after starting an SGLT-2 inhibitor) determines whether the target has been reached or another class of drugs needs to be added.

Table 3.7. Effect of Renal Function on SGLT-2 Inhibitor Doses

Drugs	Doses (mg) q.d.	eGFR (mL/min) considerations
Canagliflozin (Invokana)	100, 300	<45: both doses contraindicated 45–60: 300 mg contraindicated
Dapagliflozin (Farxiga)	5, 10	<60: both doses contraindicated; otherwise can use both doses
Empagliflozin (Jardiance)	10, 25	<45: both doses contraindicated; otherwise can use both doses

α-GLUCOSIDASE INHIBITORS

α-Glucosidases are the enzymes that break down carbohydrates to glucose, which is then absorbed from the small intestine into the circulation. Therefore, inhibition of these enzymes delays the absorption of glucose until further down in the small intestine, which in turn flattens out the postprandial rise of blood glucose concentrations.

Principles of use

Two α-glucosidase inhibitors are approved by the FDA: acarbose (Precose, Glucobay) and miglitol (Glyset). The recommended initial dose for both is 25 mg given orally at the start (with the first bite) of each main meal, and the dosage is gradually increased. However, some patients may benefit by starting at 25 mg once daily to minimize GI adverse effects (see "Adverse Effects" below) and gradually increasing the frequency of administration to three times a day before each meal. In that case, either drug should be started at 25 mg with a meal for 1–2 weeks, increased to 25 mg with a second meal for another 1–2 weeks, and finally increased to 25 mg with the third meal if the GI side effects can be tolerated by the patient. If the level of control is unsatisfactory, the dose is gradually increased to 50 mg before each meal (GI side effects permitting). Although the largest impact of the α-glucosidase inhibitors is seen on the 1- to 2-h postprandial glucose concentration, this test may be difficult to schedule accurately and is greatly influenced by the carbohydrate content of the meal. Therefore, one value may not accurately represent the patient's glycemic status. An A1C level 3 months after reaching a stable dose can be used to decide whether to continue to increase the dose. The maximal dose in patients weighing >60 kg is 100 mg three times a day and is 50 mg three times a day in patients weighing <60 kg. Alternatively, the dose can be increased gradually to the maximum (or maximally tolerated) to derive its greatest benefit in keeping with the principle of quickly determining if another drug should be added. Increasing progressively to the maximum (or maximally tolerated) dose is preferable, in our view, because if one has to wait 3 months after a submaximal dose is stabilized to evaluate the glycemic status with an A1C level, it may take up to 1 year with gradually increasing doses to determine whether an α-glucosidase inhibitor will be effective enough.

Adverse effects

The major side effect is flatulence, although a few patients may also have diarrhea. These side effects will decrease over time, especially if small doses are used initially and increased slowly, as described above. Approximately 20% of patients will have persistent flatulence and may not be able to tolerate the drug. Elevation of hepatic transaminases (ALT, AST) may rarely occur. These abnormalities are almost always reversible when the drug is discontinued. The drug is not recommended to be used in patients with intestinal disorders or in those with creatinine concentrations of >2 mg/dL (because no long-term trials in diabetes patients with this level of renal insufficiency have been conducted).

Hypoglycemia. The α-glucosidase inhibitors *will not* cause hypoglycemia when used as monotherapy. Hypoglycemia may occur, however, when the drug is added to an SU or insulin. In this case, the hypoglycemia is due, of course, to one of the latter drugs. If this should occur, *hypoglycemia must be treated with either dextrose (glucose) tablets, honey, or milk.*[65] The α-glucosidase inhibitors do not inhibit the enzyme that breaks down the carbohydrate in milk (i.e., lactose to glucose and galactose, which is why lactose intolerance is not an adverse effect of the drugs). However, these drugs will delay the absorption of other disaccharides and more complex carbohydrates, which is why these sources of carbohydrate should not be used to treat hypoglycemia. Because glucose is a monosaccharide, its absorption is not affected by α-glucosidase inhibitors.

AMYLIN MIMETICS

Amylin is co-secreted with insulin from the pancreatic β-cell. Amylin self-aggregates (sticks together to form clumps) and adheres to surfaces. By changing several amino acids in its structure, the resulting molecule (pramlintide) does not self-aggregate and is much easier with which to work. Although the physiological function of amylin is unknown, pramlintide (Symlin) has many of the properties of GLP-1. It suppresses glucagon secretion, slows gastric emptying, and decreases appetite (but does not stimulate insulin secretion).

Clinical use

Pramlintide is injected (in a separate syringe at sites at least 2 inches away from the insulin injection site) at mealtimes in patients with type 1 diabetes and insulin-requiring type 2 diabetes patients. Although there is a small significant effect on lowering FPG concentrations, as with GLP-1 agonists, its major effect is on postprandial glucose levels. Likewise, many patients also lose weight. The initial dose in type 1 diabetic patients is 15 µg before each major meal. Because of the possibility of nausea (see "Adverse Effects"), the insulin dose should be reduced by 50% and adjusted upward as indicated by glucose monitoring. If there is no significant nausea with 15 µg before each meal, the pramlintide dose is increased by 15-µg increments before each meal every 3–7 days until preprandial doses of 60 µg are reached. In insulin-requiring type 2 diabetic patients, the insulin dose is also decreased by 50% (and adjusted upward as dictated by glucose monitoring), but the initial dose of pramlintide is 60 µg before each major meal and increased in one step to maximal doses of 120 µg, nausea permitting.

Adverse effects

Approximately one-third of patients will experience significant nausea, which usually improves over time. It often reoccurs after each dose increase, but in the clinical trials, <10% withdrew because of nausea. (Note, however, that these subjects are especially motivated, and nausea may be more of a problem in the real-world setting.) In the clinical trials in which insulin doses were not changed initially, hypoglycemia was an issue, which is why an initial dose decrease of insulin (with subsequent upward titration as indicated) is recommended.

BILE ACID SEQUESTRANTS

Colesevelam (Welchol) is the only bile acid sequestrant approved for treating glycemia in diabetes. It binds bile acids in the intestinal tract, which increases bile acid production. In studies in which colesevelam has been added to metformin, an SU, or insulin, A1C levels have fallen by approximately 0.5% in patients with baseline values in the mid-7% range. The mechanism for its glycemic effect is unclear. It is supplied as a 625-mg tablet or either a 3.75-g or 1.875-g packet for oral suspension. The dose is either three tablets b.i.d. (usually with lunch and supper) or six tablets with the largest meal of the day (lunch or supper). The dose of the oral suspension is either the 1.875-g packet b.i.d (usually with lunch and supper) or one 3.75-g packet with the largest meal (lunch or supper). Because it also binds several drugs (e.g., phenytoin, warfarin, thyroid hormone, and ethinyl estradiol and nor-ethindrone in oral contraceptive agents), colesevelam should be taken at least 4 hours after these drugs. This is the reason for the recommendation for it to be taken with lunch and/or supper. Colesevelam may also decrease the absorption of the fat-soluble vitamins (A, D, E, and K). Conversely, blood metformin levels may be higher after taking its extended-release tablet. Its major adverse effects are constipation and dyspepsia, although these are alleged to be less than with the other bile acid sequestrants. An obvious advantage to colesevelam is a lowering of both cholesterol and glycemia levels, although triglyceride levels increase.

DOPAMINE-2 AGONIST

A quick-release formulation of bromocriptine (Cycloset) must be taken within 2 hours after waking (with food to avoid GI side effects). The drug works centrally to suppress the dopaminergic and sympathetic tone in the hypothalamus, resulting in decreased postprandial glucose, free fatty acid, and triglyceride levels.[66] It is marketed as a 0.8-mg tablet, which is the initial dose. The dose is increased weekly by one tablet until a maximally tolerated dose of 1.6–4.8 mg is achieved. Adverse effects include nausea, fatigue, dizziness, vomiting, and headache. Orthostatic hypotension and somnolence can also occur. The drug should be used with caution in patients with a psychotic disorder. The drug's glycemic effect is modest; in some of the clinical trials, the major A1C changes were an increase in the placebo group compared with no or only a small change in the Cycloset group. On the other hand, in a large safety trial, Cycloset was associated with a statistically significant benefit in decreasing ASCVD outcomes.[67]

TREATMENT OF MARKEDLY SYMPTOMATIC, NEWLY DIAGNOSED PATIENTS WITH TYPE 2 DIABETES

First, markedly symptomatic patients are defined here as individuals with increased urination and thirst occurring every several hours, day and night, and are often associated with weight loss in the presence of increased appetite, blurring of vision, and sometimes fungal infections. Patients recently diagnosed with type 2 diabetes can be successfully treated with maximal (<65 years of age) or half-maximal (≥65 years of age) doses of an SU.[19-21] In our experience, this therapy has been effective in >95% of over 300 such patients with type 2 diabetes, even though in some cases, their glucose levels can exceed 500 mg/dL, and they can be ketotic, some with bicarbonate levels as low as 15 mEq/L. Of course, insulin therapy is also appropriate in these patients, but using maximal doses of an SU is much easier for patients and physicians alike and just as effective in almost all cases. If these are truly recently diagnosed patients with type 2 diabetes, they will start to respond, at least to some extent, to a maximal dose of an SU within 1–2 weeks. These markedly symptomatic patients have had weeks to months of marked hyperglycemia so that another several weeks before they are brought under control will not have any long-term effects. It must be emphasized that this approach applies only to newly (or recently, within the past 6 months or so) diagnosed patients. Patients with a longer duration of diagnosed type 2 diabetes will often not have enough insulin secretion left to respond sufficiently to an insulin secretagogue.

Second, clinical clues suggesting that the patient has type 2 diabetes are *a*) obese (BMI ≥30 kg/m²) or at least overweight (BMI 26.0–29.9 kg/m²), *b*) ethnic minority, and *c*) positive family history in one or more first-degree relatives. If patients meet these criteria, especially the third one, it is likely that they have type 2 diabetes.

Third, Figure 3.4 describes the therapeutic approach used in these patients. Metformin is not used initially at maximal doses in place of an SU because high doses are likely to cause GI side effects, and the drug should be titrated up slowly to minimize these. Increasing doses of metformin often facilitates lowering the

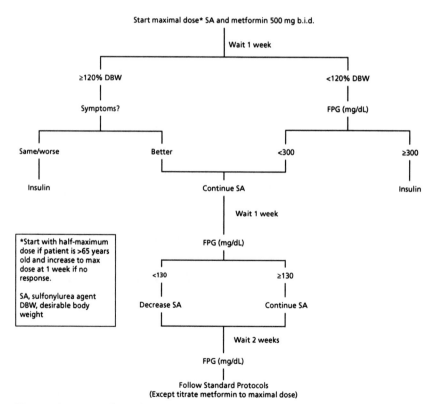

Figure 3.4. Flow diagram for treatment of markedly symptomatic, newly diagnosed type 2 diabetic patients.

SU dose, and in many cases, in these newly diagnosed patients with type 2 diabetes, the SU can be discontinued and the patient maintained on metformin alone.

Fourth, principles of the SU therapy are as follows: Most physicians start insulin in these patients, although this is rarely necessary. In those few patients who do not respond adequately to high doses of an SU and progressively increasing doses of metformin, other classes of drugs (including insulin) may then become necessary. If insulin is required, it can be started several weeks to several months later under less "emergent" conditions.

COMBINATION PILLS

A number of the oral medications and two containing insulin plus another injectable GLP-1 agonist to treat type 2 diabetes have been combined into one medication (Table 3.8). The advantages of the combinations are that they decrease the (often-large) number of medications that diabetes patients must take, and since copays are charged per medication prescribed, they are reduced as well. The disadvantages are that it can be more difficult to up-titrate the dose(s) of each drug, and combination medications are often more expensive (for the medical care system and patients via higher copays) than if each were prescribed singly. Each situation must be judged separately, but once stable doses of both drugs given separately have been reached, combination pills may be helpful for some patients.

Table 3.8. Combination Medications

Name of pill	Drug 1	Drug 2
Actoplusmet	Pioglitazone 15 mg	Metformin 500 mg
	Pioglitazone 15 mg	Metformin 850 mg
Actoplusmet XR	Pioglitazone 15 mg	Metformin extended release 1,000 mg
	Pioglitazone 30 mg	Metformin extended release 1,000 mg
Avandamet	Rosiglitazone 2 mg	Metformin 500 mg
	Rosiglitazone 4 mg	Metformin 500 mg
	Rosiglitazone 2 mg	Metformin 1,000 mg
	Rosiglitazone 4 mg	Metformin 1,000 mg
Avandaryl	Rosiglitazone 4 mg	Glimepiride 1 mg
	Rosiglitazone 4 mg	Glimepiride 2 mg
	Rosiglitazone 4 mg	Glimepiride 4 mg
	Rosiglitazone 8 mg	Glimepiride 2 mg
	Rosiglitazone 8 mg	Glimepiride 4 mg
Duetact	Pioglitazone 30 mg	Glimepiride 2 mg
	Pioglitazone 30 mg	Glimepiride 4 mg
Glucovance	Glyburide 1.25 mg	Metformin 250 mg
	Glyburide 2.5 mg	Metformin 500 mg
	Glyburide 5 mg	Metformin 500 mg

(continued on page 72)

Table 3.8. Combination Medications *(continued)*

Name of pill	Drug 1	Drug 2
Glyxambi	Empaglifloxin 10 mg	Linagliptin 5 mg
	Empaglifloxin 25 mg	Linagliptin 5 mg
Invokamet	Canagliflozin 50 mg	Metformin 500 mg
	Canagliflozin 50 mg	Metformin 1,000 mg
	Canagliflozin 150 mg	Metformin 500 mg
	Canagliflozin 150 mg	Metformin 1,000 mg
Janumet	Sitagliptin 50 mg	Metformin 500 mg
Janumet XR	Sitagliptin 50 mg	Metformin extended release 500 mg
	Sitagliptin 50 mg	Metformin extended release 1,000 mg
	Sitagliptin 100 mg	Metformin extended release 1,000 mg
Jentaducto	Linagliptin 2.5 mg	Metformin 500 mg
	Linagliptin 2.5 mg	Metformin 850 mg
	Linagliptin 2.5 mg	Metformin 1,000 mg
Kazano	Alogliptin 12.5 mg	Metformin 500 mg
	Alogliptin 12.5 mg	Metformin 1,000 mg
Kombiglyze	Saxagliptin 2.5 mg	Metformin extended release 1,000 mg
	Saxagliptin 5 mg	Metformin extended release 500 mg
	Saxagliptin 5 mg	Metformin extended release 1,000 mg
Metaglip	Glipizide 2.5 mg	Metformin 250 mg
	Glipizide 2.5 mg	Metformin 500 mg
	Glipizide 5 mg	Metformin 500 mg
Prandimet	Replaginide 1 mg	Metformin 500 mg
	Replaginide 2 mg	Metformin 500 mg
Soliqua 100/33	Glargine U-100 (100 units/mL)	Lixisenatide 33 µg/mL
Synjardy	Empagliflozin 5 mg	Metformin 500 mg
	Empagliflozin 5 mg	Metformin 1,000 mg
	Empagliflozin 12.5 mg	Metformin 500 mg
	Empagliflozin 12.5 mg	Metformin 1,000 mg
Synjardy XR	Empagliflozin 5 mg	Metformin extended release 500 mg
	Empagliflozin 5 mg	Metformin extended release 1,000 mg
	Empagliflozin 12.5 mg	Metformin extended release 500 mg
	Empagliflozin 12.5 mg	Metformin extended release 1,000 mg
Xigduo	Dapagliflozin 5 mg	Metformin 850 mg
	Dapagliflozin 5 mg	Metformin 1,000 mg
Xigduo XR	Dapagliflozin 5 mg	Metformin extended release 500 mg
	Dapagliflozin 5 mg	Metformin extended release 1,000 mg
	Dapagliflozin 10 mg	Metformin extended release 500 mg
	Dapagliflozin 10 mg	Metformin extended release 1,000 mg
Xultophy 100/3.6	Degludec U-100 (100 units/mL)	Liraglutide 3.6 mg/mL

SELF-MONITORING OF BLOOD GLUCOSE

SMBG is extremely important for adjusting insulin doses, and its use will be described in some detail in the insulin sections below. However, there is little evidence demonstrating that SMBG in non–insulin-treated patients improves glycemia. A few observational studies show that SMBG in these patients is associated with slightly lower A1C levels than in individuals who did not perform SMBG. However, this association is likely due to patient self-selection, i.e., individuals with healthier lifestyles are more likely to test,[68] or to physician self-selection, i.e., they are more likely to order SMBG in newly diagnosed patients with type 2 diabetes in whom initial treatment always improves glycemia. Figure 3.5 shows a negative correlation between A1C levels and the number of SMBG tests performed per day in patients with type 2 diabetes who require insulin, as might be expected, but also shows a positive correlation in patients not taking insulin. The latter is related to another aspect of physician self-selection, in that patients uncontrolled in the years after diagnosis are more likely to be asked to carry out more testing to bring them under control. Causation needs to be evaluated in randomized clinical trials; observational studies can only be hypothesis-generating.

Randomized control trials (RCTs) do not support the use of SMBG in non–insulin-treated diabetes patients for improving glycemia. A review of 16 RCTs revealed 11 negative studies, and in all five of the trials showing a significant low-

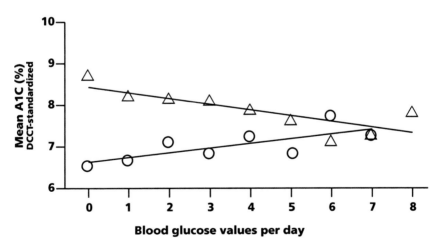

Figure 3.5. Effect of SMBG in patients with type 2 diabetes treated with insulin ($\triangle$, n = 2,021) or with oral antidiabetes drugs and/or diet ($\bigcirc$, n = 2,988). Data are adjusted for age, diabetes duration, sex, BMI–z-score, treatment center, and year of therapy. DCCT, Diabetes Control and Complications Trial. Reprinted with permission from Schutt et al.[69]

ering of A1C levels in patients performing SMBG compared with control subjects, the SMBG group received more intensive education and/or treatment than the control group.[70] Meta-analyses[71] and pooled analyses[72] of RCTs revealed a 0.25% and 0.26% difference, respectively, between SMBG and control groups after 6 months, a difference that does not meet the generally agreed, clinically relevant change of 0.5% and only 0.1% after 12 months.[72] Moreover, some patients who test have increased anxiety and depression.[72]

With a little reflection, it is not surprising that SMBG has not improved glycemic outcomes in non–insulin-treated patients. For SMBG to be helpful, patients must act on the results. Patients taking insulin can adjust their preprandial doses. For non–insulin-treated patients, only adjusting doses of a glinide or an α-glucosidase inhibitor (each of which has only ~1% market share of oral antidiabetes drugs in the U.S.) will have an effect. Patients could change the carbohydrate content or delay the meal or engage in increased exercise after the meal. However, these behavioral changes are either not being done or are ineffective (probably the former), as evidenced by the negative results of the randomized clinical trials in non–insulin-treated patients.

SMBG has been shown to be clinically effective if values are transmitted to providers frequently (every 1–4 weeks), who then increase pharmacological therapy based on these results.[73-76] This result is consistent with the critical importance of timely and appropriate therapeutic decisions to reach target levels.[77] Unfortunately, this approach is the exception to the usual quarterly office visits of patients.

SMBG has the potential to educate and motivate non–insulin-treated patients. SMBG values could educate patients on the effects of the carbohydrate content and size of meals, and high values could motivate them to follow prescribed diets and to change a sedentary lifestyle to a more active one. To maximize the education, patients should perform SMBG before and between 1 and 2 h after the same meal to isolate the glycemic response to that meal. For motivational purposes, postprandial values (preferably after the largest meal) should be measured. Regrettably, the overwhelming majority of tests in these patients are preprandial ones, usually fasting, which would have much less effect on educating and motivating patients. A more fundamental barrier for SMBG to improve glycemia in non–insulin-treated patients is the general difficulty of people changing their behaviors. To that point, there are little changes in dietary intake after people are diagnosed with diabetes.[78]

SMBG is very expensive.[79] In the absence of much evidence attesting to its benefit in patients not taking insulin, it is not part of our treatment algorithms for such patients. In a study in which a nurse treated over 350 patients in a county clinic by following these algorithms and achieved a mean A1C level of 7.0%,[80] the mean A1C level in subjects not taking insulin who also did not perform SMBG was 6.7%. Therefore, SMBG is not necessary to reach the ADA goal in non–insulin-treated patients as long as timely and appropriate treatment decisions are being made.[77]

INSULIN

The general approach in using insulin is to craft an insulin regimen around the patient's usual eating and exercise patterns rather than to impose an insulin regimen that requires patients to change their lifestyle to accommodate it. (This is not to say that one should not try to change the patient's lifestyle to a more healthy one, but one has to base the insulin regimen on what the patient is actually doing, not on what one hopes that they will do to maximize the success of insulin therapy.) From the patient's perspective, this requires a relatively consistent eating (and exercise) pattern. (Carbohydrate counting is an exception and will be discussed below.) This approach can sometimes be quite challenging, e.g., in patients who work evening or overnight shifts during the week but not on weekends. But in the final analysis, this approach is the only way for these patients to control their glycemia without having diabetes markedly disrupt their lives. The following five questions should be asked of all insulin-treated patients when adjusting their doses:

1. What are the insulins and their doses currently being taken? The reason for this question is obvious.
2. What are the frequency of SMBG and the pattern of the resultant glucose values? When is SMBG being carried out and how often at each time? Preprandial and before-bedtime snack are the usual times recommended in patients taking two or more injections of insulin a day, whereas only FPG measurements are necessary in patients taking basal insulin alone or bedtime NPH insulin alone. (We recommend that every patient taking insulin should take a small bedtime snack to minimize overnight hypoglycemia; see below for more details.) If all preprandial values are on-target, and the A1C level is still above target (usually >7.0%), 1- to 2-h postprandial glucose concentrations should be measured. In that case, these postprandial tests substitute for the subsequent preprandial tests, e.g., postprandial breakfast tests replace the preprandial lunch tests, which should be in the target range before asking for postprandial testing.
3. What are the glucose values at each time of testing? As discussed below, the results at each time reflect a different component of the insulin prescription. Therefore, daily, weekly, or monthly average values throughout the day are not helpful in adjusting insulin doses.
4. What are the frequency and patterns of hypoglycemia? If hypoglycemia occurs less than once or twice a month, it probably does not need to be specifically addressed. If it occurs more frequently, its pattern (i.e., when it occurs) may give a clue as to how to address it. For example, if hypoglycemia usually occurs between breakfast and lunch, the dose of short- or rapid-acting insulin taken before breakfast needs to be decreased. Hypoglycemia occurring overnight may necessitate starting a bedtime snack (if that is not already part of the patient's usual eating pattern); reducing the evening NPH, or basal insulin dose; or possibly moving the NPH injection from before supper to bedtime.
5. Is hypoglycemia explained or unexplained? This is extremely important to differentiate. *Explained* hypoglycemia occurs if a meal is delayed or missed or unanticipated exercise takes place, or occasionally if a higher-than-prescribed dose of insulin is taken. Consistency of lifestyle needs to be stressed in this case. *Unexplained* hypoglycemia occurs in the presence of the patient's usual eating and exercise patterns. In this case, the appropriate insulin dose needs to be adjusted downward.

Many patients will state that they have had episodes of (undocumented) hypoglycemia. It is important for the provider to determine whether these are bona fide hypoglycemic episodes. In addition to deciding whether the symptoms are consistent with hypoglycemia, the key questions to ask are whether the patient ate something at that time to treat it, and if so, how long it took to feel better. If the symptoms don't start to improve within 20 minutes (often much faster) after eating, it is unlikely that this represents true hypoglycemia.

Severe hypoglycemia is defined as an episode that requires third-party assistance to treat, i.e., the patient is unable to recognize the symptoms and take appropriate measures to reverse it. If this is an unexplained occurrence, it needs to be addressed by changing the appropriate insulin dose regardless of its frequency. Explained episodes of severe hypoglycemia require intense education to identify for the patient the circumstances that led to it. The sometimes difficult issue of hypoglycemia and driving is nicely covered by the ADA in the Clinical Practice Recommendations.[81]

INSULIN PREPARATIONS

Most insulin preparations are U-100, which means that there are 100 units per mL. Neutral Protamine Hagedorn (NPH) and regular insulins are human insulins. All of the others are analog insulins, in which their structures have been changed, and in some cases, they have been bound to other molecules, both of which alter their pharmacokinetic and pharmacodynamic properties. Clinically, there is little difference between human and analog insulins. There is no difference in their effectiveness, but there is a slight, yet statistically significant, decrease in overnight hypoglycemia with analog basal insulins compared to bedtime NPH insulin[82] and with degludec insulin compared with glargine[83] and detemir[84] insulins. Most insulin preparations are also available in pens, which are much more convenient than using insulin vials, syringes, and needles. The terminology of the many insulin preparations is shown in Table 3.9.

The pharmacokinetic and pharmacodynamic properties of the various types of insulin are described in Table 3.10. The times shown are approximate. There is a

Table 3.9. Terminology of Insulin Preparations

- Short-acting (Regular): Humulin R; Novolin R; Relion R (only available at Walmart)
- Rapid-acting: Lispro (Humalog*); Aspart (Novolog); Glulisine (Apidra); Afrezza (inhaled)
- Intermediate-acting (NPH): Humulin N; Novolin N; Relion N (Walmart) N; Humulin R U-500†
- Basal (peakless): Glargine (Lantus, Tuojeo‡, Basaglar); Detemir (Levemir); Degludec (Tresiba*)
- Premixed: Novolin 70/30 (70% NPH/30% regular); Humulin 70/30 (70% NPH/30% regular); Novolog Mix 70/30 (70% aspart protamine suspension/30% aspart); Humalog Mix 75/25 (75% lispro protamine suspension/25% lispro); Humalog Mix 50/50 (50% lispro protamine suspension/50% lispro); Ryzodeg 70/30 (70% degludec/30% aspart)

*Both U-100 and U-200 (200 units per mL); †U-500 (500 units of regular insulin per mL, which has a time course of action similar to NPH insulin but with little acute postprandial effect); ‡U-300 (300 units per mL).

Table 3.10. Time Course of Action of Insulins

Insulin	Onset (hours)	Peak (hours)	Duration (hours)
Short-acting	0.5–1.0	2–4	4–6
Rapid-acting	0.15–0.25	1–2	~3
Intermediate-acting (NPH)	3–4	6–12	~18
Intermediate-acting (U-500 regular)	0.5–1.0	7–9	~12
Basal (peakless) Glargine Detemir Degludec	Not applicable		~24 ~20 ~40
Premixed	Combination of individual components		

20–30% intra-individual variability from day to day in a person's response to insulin.[85,86] This, plus the variability in eating patterns, is the reason why insulin doses should be adjusted on patterns of glucose values rather than on just a few numbers. These variabilities explain why the older teaching that regular insulin should be injected 20–30 minutes before a meal is unnecessary. A cross-over study comparing injecting regular insulin 20 minutes and immediately before eating revealed identical mean pre- and postprandial SMBG values for the subsequent 6 weeks.[87]

PRINCIPLES OF ADJUSTING INSULIN DOSES

Although there is no one "right" way to use insulin, there are some important principles and relationships that underlie the appropriate use of insulin. Table 3.11 describes the most important relationships among various components of the insulin regimens, their injection times, the periods of the day/night that they maximally cover, and the most appropriate SMBG tests to judge their effects.

Preprandial testing is preferred because it is much easier for patients to remember and to accommodate this activity when they are stopping for a meal (and usually an insulin injection) rather than remembering to stop what they are doing 1–2 hours after eating to perform the test. However, as described above, if preprandial values are at target and the A1C levels remain too high, postprandial testing is indicated to determine if high glucose levels after meals (with return to target levels before the next meal) may explain the above-target A1C levels.

Each component of the insulin prescription is changed (or not) depending on the pattern of results of SMBG tests that reflects its maximal activity. How should this be done? First, one must decide on the appropriate target ranges for each of these times. The ADA in 2015 changed its recommended preprandial target range of 70–130 mg/dL to 80–130 mg/dL to better reflect new data comparing actual average glucose levels with A1C targets.[1] However, using this preprandial target range suggests that glucose values of 70–79 mg/dL are hypoglycemic, which contradicts the previous ADA definition of hypoglycemia as <70 mg/dL.[88] Therefore, we continue to use the older preprandial target range of 70–130 mg/dL. The ADA

Table 3.11. Relationships Among Components of Various Insulin Regimens, Times of Injection, Periods of Maximal Effects, and Tests to Judge Effects

Insulin	When injected	Period covered	Tests best reflecting effect
Short-acting	Before breakfast	Morning	After breakfast/before lunch
Rapid-acting	Before breakfast	Morning	After breakfast/before lunch
Intermediate-acting	Before breakfast	Afternoon	After lunch/before supper
Basal	Before breakfast	Overnight	Before breakfast
Short-acting	Before lunch	Afternoon	After lunch/before supper
Rapid-acting	Before lunch	Afternoon	After lunch/before supper
Short-acting	Before supper	Evening	After supper/before bedtime (snack)
Rapid-acting	Before supper	Evening	After supper/before bedtime (snack)
Intermediate-acting	Before supper/bedtime	Overnight	Before breakfast
Basal	Bedtime	Overnight	Before breakfast
Basal	Half before breakfast/half before bedtime	Overnight	Before breakfast
Premixed*	Before breakfast	Morning/afternoon	After breakfast/before lunch and after lunch/before supper
Premixed*	Before supper	Evening/overnight	After supper/before bedtime (snack) and before breakfast
Ryzodeg	Before breakfast	Morning/overnight	After breakfast/before lunch and before breakfast next day
Ryzodeg	Before supper	Evening/overnight	After supper/before bedtime (snack) and before breakfast

*With the exception of Ryzodeg.

kept its previous postprandial target of <180 mg/dL 1–2 hours after eating.[1] We feel that this postprandial target is too high; instead, we use a postprandial target range of 100–160 mg/dL, which also differs from the ADA by defining a lower target as well.

The next step is to decide under what circumstances changes in insulin doses should be made. If a test at a specific time of day (usually before a meal or the bedtime snack) is consistently too high, i.e., higher than the upper limit of the target range, or too low, i.e., less than the lower limit of the target range, raise or lower the appropriate insulin dose by 2 units in lean patients, by 4 units in overweight/obese patients, or by 10% of the current dose (whichever is higher). Larger dose increases may be in order if glucose values are "very high," e.g., >70 mg/dL above the upper limit of the target range. If 50% or more of the high values are "very high," insulin doses could be raised by 4 units in lean patients, by 8 units in overweight/obese patients, or by 15% of the current dose (whichever is higher).

For insulin dose adjustments, we designate individuals as overweight/obese if they are ≥120% of their desirable body weight (DBW). This value was selected because life expectancy starts to decrease at weights exceeding this level. The calculation of DBW[89] is described in Table 2.1. Alternatively, one could use BMI for the designation of overweight/obese. We would suggest using the older BMI definition of obesity of ≥27 kg/m² to define overweight/obese because it captures the upper cohort of the current BMI definition of overweight (25.1–29.9 kg/m²).

Glucose concentrations at a specific time are "too high" if the number of values that exceed the upper target level *minus* the number of values that are less than the lower target level *plus* the number of bona fide episodes of *unexplained* hypoglycemia, for which no measured low glucose levels are available, constitute 50% or more of the glucose concentrations during that postprandial/preprandial time of day (Table 3.11) during the dates being considered. As examples, that would be on ≥2 of 3 days, ≥4 of 7 days, ≥5 of 10 days, ≥7 of 14 days, ≥11 of 21 days, ≥14 of 28 days, ≥18 of 35 days, ≥21 of 42 days, or ≥50% of the values during any number of days between 1 and 6 weeks.

Conversely, the glucose concentrations at a specific time are "too low" if the number of values that are less than the lower target level *plus* the number of bona fide episodes of *unexplained* hypoglycemia, for which no measured low glucose levels are available, *minus* the number of values that exceed the upper target level constitute 50% or more of the glucose concentrations at that time of day during a 1- to 6-week period.

If the glucose concentrations at a specific time of day are neither "too high" nor "too low," no change is made in that component of the insulin prescription that primarily affects the test at that time of day. We prefer to analyze SMBG results at least every 6 weeks once insulin doses are reasonably stable because over longer periods, patients (at least the minority ones that we serve) often become less adherent to the recommended insulin doses and SMBG testing frequency.

No adjustment is made in that component of the insulin prescription for which the number of appropriate tests is too few. The way to judge "too few" is to decide how many SMBG values at the particular time of day/overnight during the number of days being evaluated would be necessary before a decision should be made on the dose of that component of the insulin regimen that maximally affects that period. We would suggest that at least one-third and preferably up to one-half of the days being evaluated have SMBG values during the period of time that maximally reflects the component of the insulin regimen that is being considered for a dose adjustment. Fewer values might not accurately reflect the usual eating/exercise pattern of the patient.

The desired frequency of daily SMBG testing for insulin dose adjustments is another important issue. Patients taking bedtime NPH insulin alone or only one of the basal insulins need only test before breakfast. Once two or more insulin injections are required, testing before each meal and the bedtime snack would be ideal. However, it is usually unrealistic to expect this degree of testing for most patients. We strongly recommend that patients test at least twice a day, alternating before breakfast and before supper with before lunch and before the bedtime snack.

We even more strongly recommend that all patients taking insulin ingest a small bedtime snack containing some protein to decrease the chances of overnight hypoglycemia. In our practice, it is unusual for patients taking a bedtime snack to experience overnight hypoglycemia. Patients are instructed to decrease their supper calories to accommodate the bedtime ones. Even if they should gain a few pounds, the additional cardiovascular risk in these obese individuals is minimal, especially compared with avoiding a potentially serious episode of overnight hypoglycemia. For example, the increase in the risk of cardiovascular disease in a 250-lb patient who may gain 10 more pounds is minimal. On the other hand, patients experiencing hypoglycemia, especially if occurring overnight, may be reluctant to increase their insulin doses when necessary. Some simply discontinue insulin altogether, and convincing them to restart it may be difficult.

Hypoglycemia is another important factor affecting insulin dose adjustments. Frankly, few patients perform SMBG when they are experiencing hypoglycemia; treating it typically overrides testing. Therefore, deciding whether the episode described is bona fide hypoglycemia or not is an important issue for making insulin dose adjustments. Readers of this volume will certainly be familiar with the symptoms of hypoglycemia, but as is well known, a number of the symptoms are nonspecific. If the provider is fairly certain that the episode was indeed a hypoglycemic one, the next step is to ascertain whether it was explained or unexplained as discussed above. Bona fide episodes of unexplained episodes are included in the analysis (even though no glucose documentation has occurred); education is (again) stressed for the explained ones. Often patients will test after starting to treat the episode to determine if more carbohydrate is necessary. These results (often high because of overtreatment) should be ignored in the analysis.

When to initiate insulin therapy

Patients with type 1 diabetes, of course, need insulin immediately after diagnosis. An exception is patients with latent autoimmune diabetes of the adult (LADA) who may be controlled on noninsulin medications for a while (although for a much shorter period than patients with type 2 diabetes). Because of the difficulties of using insulin (from both the patient and provider perspectives), as long as patients with LADA meet A1C targets, we do not use insulin. As soon as noninsulin medications fail, insulin is started. Although many guidelines recommend insulin in patients with type 2 diabetes with high A1C levels, this treatment is not always necessary. Asymptomatic newly diagnosed patients will usually respond to metformin alone, and for those who do not at the maximal (tolerated) dose, adding an SU (or another noninsulin medication) will almost always enable them to reach target A1C levels. Almost all markedly symptomatic, newly diagnosed patients (irrespective of their glucose and A1C levels) will respond quickly to maximal doses of an SU,[19-21] with reduction of the initial dose often necessary to avoid hypoglycemia as described previously. This approach avoids the hassles of starting insulin, the frequent down-titration, and the not uncommon discontinuation of insulin that occurs in patients with newly diagnosed type 2 diabetes. On the other hand, because of the progressive loss of insulin secretion in type 2 diabetes, patients with a long duration and very high A1C levels do require insulin.

Bedtime NPH and basal insulin regimens

Almost all patients with type 2 diabetes (with the exception of newly diagnosed individuals in whom insulin may have been [unnecessarily] initiated) will have been treated with a combination of two to four noninsulin medications before insulin is started. Several older studies have shown that when patients failed maximal doses of metformin plus an SU, multiple-dose insulin regimens did not yield better control than bedtime NPH insulin plus oral anti-diabetes drugs when compared for up to 1 year.[90–93] Therefore, if the FPG concentration can be lowered appreciably, overall diabetic control is often significantly improved (Figure 3.6).

Bedtime NPH or a basal insulin is an easy way to introduce insulin therapy to patients with type 2 diabetes who have failed noninsulin drugs. There is only one insulin injection, and initially, it is necessary to measure only the FPG level. Because the peak effect of the NPH insulin occurs around breakfast time and glargine, detemir, and degludec insulins are peakless, there is much less chance of daytime hypoglycemia mediated by exogenous insulin compared to a regimen in which NPH insulin is injected before breakfast or short- or rapid-acting insulin is given before meals. Bedtime NPH or basal insulin gives patients much more flexibility in their eating and exercise patterns during the day. As mentioned previously, there are somewhat fewer overnight hypoglycemic reactions with glargine, detemir, and degludec insulin compared with NPH insulin and fewer with degludec compared with glargine and detemir. (However, we have had little difficulty with overnight hypoglycemia using *gradual* increases in the doses of NPH and basal insulin, especially when the patient ingests a small bedtime snack.)

Although the ADA A1C target is <7.0% in most patients, insulin is not started in our practice until the A1C level exceeds 7.4% because the risk of the microvascular complications is only slightly increased between A1C levels of 7.0 and 7.5%

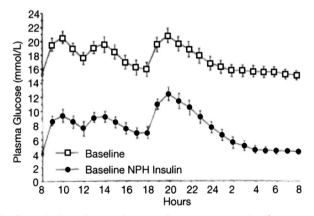

Figure 3.6. One- to two-hour plasma glucose concentrations over a 24-hour period in patients taking maximal doses of either glyburide (20 mg/day) or glipizide (40 mg/day) (upper curve) or bedtime NPH insulin without SUs (lower curve). Reprinted with permission from Cusi et al.[94]

(Figure 1.1). Also, using insulin appropriately creates changes in a person's lifestyle (e.g., injections, SMBG, and risk of hypoglycemia). For patients in which A1C targets should be less stringent,[1] we use an A1C level of ≥8.0% before introducing insulin.

Overweight and obese patients are started on 16 units and lean patients on 10 units of bedtime NPH insulin or one of the basal insulins. Alternatively, the initial dose can be calculated as 0.2 units/kg body weight. The starting insulin doses are almost always less than the patient eventually requires but do avoid overnight hypoglycemia initially, which might well discourage the patient from remaining on this therapy. The dose is increased as described above, i.e., if 50% of the SMBG values before breakfast exceed the target, the dose is raised by 4 units in overweight/obese patients and by 2 units in lean patients, or 10% of the dose (whichever is higher). Ideally, test values should be acted on frequently (every 3–7 days) when insulin is started, but as values approach target levels, longer intervals between adjustments are in order. We prefer adjusting the dose at least once a week for several weeks after starting insulin, every 2 weeks as the dose continues to be titrated upward, every 3 weeks as the dose becomes stabilized, and every 6 weeks on an ongoing basis. Of course, one's practice situation will largely determine the frequency of adjustments.

Many patients with type 2 diabetes are very obese and consequently require large doses of insulin to reach target FPG concentrations. Because this can take many months to achieve, we attempt to teach these patients to self-titrate the insulin dose based on their FPG levels. Overweight/obese and lean patients are instructed to increase their bedtime dose by 2 units and 1 unit, respectively, each evening if that morning's value exceeded 130 mg/dL. Conversely, if the value were <70 mg/dL, the dose would be decreased by that amount. Patients on high doses (>80 units) of the U-100 basal insulins are instructed to inject one-half of the dose twice a day, since large volumes of injectate can impair absorption. In that case, lean and overweight/obese patients are instructed to increase each dose of the basal insulin by 1 or 2 units, respectively. Self-titration ceases when there have been no dose changes for 1 week. Self-titration instructions for patients in English and Spanish are included in the Appendix. The provider can simply circle the appropriate information that applies to a specific patient.

Noninsulin medications and bedtime NPH or basal insulins

According to the protocols described earlier in the chapter, patients starting bedtime NPH insulin or one of the basal insulins will be taking up to four of the following noninsulin medications: metformin, an SU, a DPP-4 inhibitor, a TZD, a GLP-1 agonist, and an SGLT-2 inhibitor. With the exception of a TZD, we maintain patients on their noninsulin medications to maximize the chances that daytime glycemia will be controlled after the FPG target is reached. TZDs are discontinued because they will enhance the weight gain seen with introducing insulin, increase the degree of fluid retention, and thereby increase the risk of heart failure. One must remain cognizant that DKA can rarely occur in patients with type 2 diabetes taking insulin and an SGLT-2 inhibitor, sometimes presenting with glucose concentrations <250 mg/dL.[60]

Failure of bedtime NPH or basal insulin regimens

When should bedtime NPH or basal insulins plus daytime noninsulin drugs be judged ineffective and a multiple-dose insulin regimen be instituted? The answer is not until the target FPG concentrations are achieved and A1C levels 3 months later are too high. A common error is to give up before reaching target FPG concentrations. This scenario usually occurs in obese patients in whom not enough insulin is prescribed and the FPG levels hover around the mid to high 100s. Many of these patients are extremely obese, with resulting severe insulin resistance. They sometimes require up to 100 units or more of NPH or a basal insulin. Overnight hypoglycemia is seldom a problem because, as mentioned previously, the insulin doses are gradually increased; NPH insulin peaks around breakfast time (not in the middle of the night when given before supper); glargine, detemir, and degludec insulins are peakless; and patients are strongly encouraged to eat a small bedtime snack.

Once >50% of the SMBG values are within the FPG target range, the A1C level determines whether the bedtime NPH or basal insulin regimen is sufficient to control the patient. Because of the delay of A1C levels to plateau,[95] this decision should be made after waiting 3 months. Soon after reaching the FPG target range, there is reason to test a few times before supper. With FPG levels this much lower, the maximal dose of the SU may cause daytime hypoglycemia. Before-supper values <80 mg/dL may presage daytime hypoglycemia, and the SU dose should be halved. If before-supper values of <80 mg/dL persist, the SU should be discontinued. Of course, halving and possibly subsequently discontinuing the SU dose should also occur with bona fide unexplained episodes of (undocumented) daytime hypoglycemia as well. Conversely, once FPG levels reach the target range, before-supper glucose values that consistently exceed 180 mg/dL strongly suggest that the target A1C level of <7.5% will not be attained in 3 months hence and intensification of the insulin regimen could be considered at this point.

MULTIPLE-INJECTION INSULIN REGIMENS: GENERAL CONSIDERATIONS

We also use an A1C level ≥7.5% to signal the need to switch to two or more injections of insulin because multiple-dose insulin regimens are much more difficult for patients when followed appropriately (e.g., more frequent SMBG is required, there is more risk of hypoglycemia, especially during the daytime, and there is less flexibility with dietary and exercise patterns with two of the regimens to be considered). There are three possible intensified insulin regimens that could be used: basal/bolus, self-mixed/split, and premixed insulin. We give patients the choice of the basal/bolus or the self-mixed split regimen, explaining the pros and cons of each.

Basal/bolus insulin regimen

The basal/bolus insulin regimen usually consists of a basal insulin plus a short- or rapid-acting insulin before meals. In patients with type 2 diabetes, NPH insulin given once daily before bedtime instead of a basal insulin would also be appropriate because these patients retain some insulin secretion. NPH insulin given once daily at bedtime would not be appropriate for patients with type 1 diabetes because if there is a long period of time between lunch and supper, the effect of the before-lunch insulin injection might wane and patients would experience high before-supper glucose concentrations, since their endogenous insulin secretion is minimal. This potential problem is much more likely if a rapid-acting, rather than a short-acting, insulin is the preprandial insulin preparation used before lunch. The basal/bolus approach requires four injections of insulin, which is a problem for some patients. On the other hand, it should be strongly considered for patients with irregular eating (and exercise) patterns.

Some investigators have recommended that initially upon switching to a basal/bolus regimen, short- or rapid-acting insulin only needs to be taken before the largest meal.[96] Once the preprandial target for the following meal is reached (or before-bedtime snack if the largest meal is at supper) and the A1C remains above target, short- or rapid-acting insulin is introduced before the next largest meal. This step is repeated if the second preprandial bolus injection of short- or rapid-acting insulin achieves the subsequent preprandial target but the A1C target is still not reached. At that point, short- or rapid-acting insulin is required before all three meals.

There are two potential problems with this approach. Although logically appealing, it can lead to long delays in reaching target A1C levels. First, the target level of glucose, either postprandially or before the subsequent meal (or bedtime snack in case supper is the meal in question), must be achieved. Then, at least a further 3 months must elapse before the A1C level will accurately reflect overall glycemia. This period will be doubled if an injection before a second meal is required and tripled if injections before all three meals are deemed necessary. Because only 22–30% of patients on basal insulins who begin a basal/bolus regimen by adding a single preprandial bolus dose achieve an A1C level of <7.0%,[97-99] there will be long delays in reaching A1C goals in the majority of these patients. Indeed, a recent study of stepwise increases in the number of preprandial injections showed that 8 months was required for the A1C levels to match those achieved in patients who were initially placed on all three preprandial injections, and only 17% remained on one bolus dose.[100]

The second potential problem is that the most important determinant of postprandial glucose concentrations (and therefore the preprandial ones before the next meal) is the starting preprandial value. The increases in postprandial glucose concentrations over preprandial values are similar regardless of the starting preprandial glucose levels.[94,101,102] Therefore, postprandial hyperglycemia is initially best treated by lowering preprandial glucose levels. In the situation where a preprandial injection before a single meal has controlled postprandial glucose concentrations after that meal but A1C levels have not reached target, a second preprandial injection must be introduced. However, when the second injection lowers the preprandial values before the initial meal that had just been successfully treated, the short- or rapid-acting insulin dose given before that first meal may be too high, leading to postprandial hypoglycemia. The same potential problem occurs when a third preprandial injection is introduced. For these two reasons, we usually start preprandial short- or rapid-acting insulin before all three meals when instituting basal/bolus regimens.

Because the current bedtime NPH or basal insulin dose has achieved the FPG target, we continue it without changing the dose. The initial preprandial short- or rapid-acting insulin dose is 2–4 units in lean patients and 6–8 units in overweight/obese patients. These doses almost always need to be increased, but starting at this level avoids hypoglycemia, which will often discourage patients from continuing this intensified regimen.

Self-mixed/split insulin regimen

In the self-mixed/split insulin regimen (mentioned only briefly[103] in the updated ADA/EASD position statement on the management of hyperglycemia[3]), the insulin preparations are mixed in the same syringe and injected twice a day. If used properly, this approach can yield as tight control as a basal/bolus regimen.[104,105] However, patients have less flexibility with their eating (and exercise) patterns with this regimen, especially with the timing of lunch and supper because of the time course of action of the before-breakfast NPH injection (Table 3.10). To switch from the bedtime NPH or basal insulin regimen, we take 80% of that dose as the total NPH dose of the self-mixed split regimen and give two-thirds before breakfast and one-third before supper. This amount is most often less than the patient will eventually require but avoids hypoglycemia, which will often discourage patients from continuing this intensified regimen. Again, to avoid hypoglycemia, the maximal initial NPH dose is 40 units before breakfast and 20 units before supper (corresponding to a bedtime NPH or total basal insulin dose of 75 units).

Since almost all patients will require short- or rapid-acting insulin to achieve the A1C target, we routinely add a small amount of one of these insulins to each NPH injection after several visits. Initially, patients are asked to perform SMBG before breakfast and before supper to adjust the NPH insulin doses. When these levels are lowered to <200 mg/dL, SMBG values before lunch and the bedtime snack are necessary to adjust the short- or rapid-acting insulin doses. Although measuring four times a day before each meal and the bedtime snack is ideal, realistically, most patients will not test this frequently. Alternatively, patients are asked to alternate their twice-a-day testing to before breakfast and supper 1 day and before lunch and the bedtime snack the next day. The latter tests allow adjusting the short- or rapid-acting insulin doses.

Only when the before-supper and before-breakfast glucose concentrations are brought down to <200 mg/dL with the appropriate NPH insulin doses are the short- or rapid-acting insulin doses increased. The reason for this is because larger doses of the short- or rapid-acting insulins will be necessary to lower the before-lunch and before-bedtime (snack) glucose concentrations to target ranges when the before-breakfast and before-supper glucose concentrations, respectively, are higher than when they are lower. For example, to reach a before-lunch glucose concentration of <130 mg/dL will require more short- or rapid-acting insulin when the FPG concentration is 250 mg/dL than when it is 120 mg/dL. Delaying the increase of the short- or rapid-acting insulin until the doses of NPH insulin have started to achieve better control reduces the possibility of hypoglycemic reactions. On the other hand, if one waits until target levels before breakfast and supper are reached before adjusting the appropriate doses of the short- or rapid-acting insulin, too much time usually elapses before control is further tightened.

Given that the peak effect of NPH insulin taken before supper occurs between 6 and 12 hours later, as one increases this dose to control the FPG concentration, hypoglycemia may occur overnight before the fasting target is reached. Decreasing the before-supper dose may well avoid the overnight hypoglycemia but will work against achieving the FPG target. If the patient is already taking a bedtime snack, that option is not available to avoid the overnight hypoglycemia. In that event, moving the NPH insulin to bedtime will almost always take care of the problem because the peak effect of the evening intermediate-acting insulin is now at breakfast time when the patient is about to eat. This change converts the two-injection self-mixed/split regimen to a three-injection regimen. However, it is often the only way to both avoid overnight hypoglycemia and meet the FPG target without converting to a basal/bolus four-injection regimen.

Determining doses of short- or rapid-acting insulins

There are two ways to decide on the usual doses of short- or rapid-acting insulin. Some more sophisticated patients can learn carbohydrate counting, and the entire preprandial dose of these insulins is based on the amount of carbohydrate to be ingested, usually 1 unit per 10–15 grams.[106] In a self-mixed/split regimen, this regimen would work for breakfast and supper, but in our view, would not be suitable for lunch. As mentioned previously, both the morning NPH insulin and the short- or rapid-acting insulin before lunch have maximal effects between lunch and supper. It would not be clear which dose of insulin to adjust in response to the pre-supper SMBG values. It would also be a third injection of insulin for the patient, negating one of the advantages of the two-injection self-mixed/split regimen.

The other dietary approach is a constant carbohydrate one in which patients are instructed on the carbohydrate content of various meal products and asked to ingest a relatively consistent amount of carbohydrate at each meal, i.e., a similar amount at each breakfast, lunch, and supper from day-to-day (not a similar amount at each meal of the day). There is no evidence that carbohydrate counting leads to better control than the constant carbohydrate dietary approach[107] (which is similar to the older "exchange system"). For patients on a fixed daily insulin schedule, the preprandial short- or rapid-acting insulin dose (in both self-mixed/split or basal/bolus regimens) can be broken down into three components. The *basic dose* is the amount prescribed to be taken before the meal and is the dose that is adjusted based on the pattern of SMBG values as described above. The *correction or supplemental dose* depends on the preprandial glucose concentration. Some patients are also able to incorporate an *anticipatory dose* that depends on anticipated meal-related issues or in the several hours after it. For instance, if patients are eating at a Chinese restaurant, they may add a few units (in addition to any correction dose) anticipating a higher carbohydrate meal than usual. Alternatively, if patients are going to engage in more exercise than usual after supper, they may reduce the short- or rapid-acting insulin dose taken before the meal that would have been dictated by the basic and correction doses. There is no formula for anticipatory doses. They must be arrived at empirically based on the patients' ongoing experiences.

In some hospitalized and nursing home patients (and in some cases those residing in a free-living environment), planned meals are incompletely ingested.

This scenario increases the chances of postprandial hypoglycemia if the prescribed dose of the short- or rapid-acting insulin is taken before the meal. If this situation keeps occuring, a rapid-acting insulin can be taken after the meal is completed without jeopardizing subsequent daily glycemia.[108] With this approach, the patient will know how much of the planned meal was actually ingested and can estimate how much to reduce the dose of the rapid-acting insulin, i.e., an "anticipatory" change occurring after the amount of the ingested meal is known. The patient should take into account any correction dose that might have been appropriate in deciding the amount of rapid-acting insulin to inject postprandially, i.e., any meal-related reduction should come from the basic dose.

Correction (supplemental) doses

Assuming no change in the carbohydrate content of the usual meal, high pre-prandial glucose concentrations require additional short- or rapid-acting insulin to lower the subsequent preprandial SMBG value into the target range. Table 3.12 shows the extra doses of these insulins we start with to *add* to (or subtract from) the basic dose to "correct" for the elevated glucose concentrations. To evaluate the responses to these corrections doses, we use a target range for the subsequent preprandial SMBG value of 100–150 mg/dL. If the majority of responses to a specific correction dose is >150 mg/dL, the correction dose needs to be increased; if the majority is <100 mg/dL (plus episodes of undocumented unexplained hypo-glycemia), it should be decreased. A minimum of three responses to a specific correction dose is necessary before it can be evaluated. For example, if there are five instances where the patient added 2 units of regular insulin for preprandial SMBG values between 201 and 250 mg/dL, and the subsequent preprandial results were >150 mg/dL on four occasions, the correction dose for this prepran-dial range would be increased to +3 units. In that case, this amount of short- or rapid-acting insulin would be added for the preprandial range of 201–300 mg/dL. If subsequent experience showed that this correction dose of +3 units was inade-quate for the preprandial range of 251–300 mg/dL, the correction dose would be increased to +4 units for this latter range of preprandial values. To simplify the

Table 3.12. Initial Correction (Supplemental) Doses of Short- or Rapid-Acting Insulin

Blood glucose (mg/dL)	Lean	Overweight/obese*
<70	–1 unit	–2 units
70–150	0 units	0 units
151–200	+1 unit	+2 units
201–250	+2 units	+4 units
251–300	+3 units	+6 units
301–350	+4 units	+8 units
>350	+5 units	+10 units

*≥120% desirable body weight (DBW) as calculated in Table 2.1.

evaluation, it is helpful if patients record the basic insulin dose and the added (or subtracted) correction dose separately, e.g., 3 + 2, units taken before the meal in a log book. Readers familiar with correction doses will note that this initial schedule suggests progressively increasing extra amounts of insulin for each 50 mg/dL above 150 mg/dL.

Premixed insulins

Although premixed insulin preparations obviate the need to have patients mix two different insulin preparations in the same syringe before injection, they have a major drawback. *One cannot adjust the doses of the intermediate-acting and short- or rapid-acting insulin separately.* For example, a common SMBG pattern in patients taking a premixed insulin preparation is high before lunch glucose concentrations but acceptable before-supper values. Raising the morning dose to lower the before-lunch levels would jeopardize the before-supper situation. Note that 70–75% of the increased before-breakfast dose will work mostly in the afternoon and only 25–30% will be available to adjust the morning hyperglycemia. Another common pattern is high before-bedtime (snack) SMBG values but acceptable before-breakfast levels. Raising the before-supper dose to lower the before-bedtime tests would facilitate overnight hypoglycemia. Therefore, achieving near-euglycemia with premixed insulins is often not possible, and these insulin preparations should be used only by patients who cannot be taught to mix insulins themselves and for whom no family or other caregiver support is available. In our experience, most patients can be taught to mix insulin, although sometimes persistent instruction is necessary.

Premixed insulins necessitate a slightly different approach than described for other insulin regimens in which each component of the regimen can be adjusted independently from other components. With the exception of the rarely used premixed insulin preparation containing 50% of intermediate-acting and 50% short- or rapid-acting insulin, other premixed insulin preparations contain 70–75% of intermediate-acting and 25–30% of short- or rapid-acting insulin. Thus, a dose increase of 4 units would deliver an additional 2.8 units of the intermediate-acting insulin and only 1.2 units of the short- or rapid-acting insulin. Therefore, dose changes of premixed insulins should be 3 and 6 units in lean and overweight/obese patients, respectively. If the glucose pattern yields "very high" readings as defined previously, the dose increase should be 6 and 10 units, respectively. Because there are two components in premixed insulin preparations, each with a maximal effect during a different time period, one must be certain that there is not a "too low" pattern in one of the time periods that would be affected by a dose increase in response to a "too high" pattern during another time period. For example, if the morning patterns were high, which would require increasing the dose of the before-breakfast premixed preparation, but the afternoon pattern was "too low," not only should the morning premixed insulin dose not be increased, it should be decreased to raise the afternoon glucose values. *Preventing hypoglycemia takes precedence.* The same dose changes could be used for the 50–50% premixed insulin preparations but realize that there would be equal effects in both of the time periods covered by those preparations.

Humulin U-500 regular insulin

It is not uncommon for very obese patients with type 2 diabetes to require hundreds of units of insulin to achieve satisfactory control. Some, in spite of testing appropriately and increasing insulin doses as recommended, are unable to achieve A1C levels <8.0% because large volumes of injectate impair insulin absorption.[109] These patients receiving a total of >200 units of U-100 insulin per day are switched to injections of Humulin U-500 regular insulin before breakfast and before supper. The time course of action of Humulin U-500 regular insulin is similar to NPH insulin.[110] Initial doses and dose adjustments are shown in Figure 3.7. If A1C levels remain ≥7.5% after the before-breakfast and before-supper SMBG values reach target levels, separate injections of short- or rapid-acting insulin are given along with the U-500 insulin. We usually start with 6 units, and inexplicably, before-lunch and before-bedtime SMBG values show that these patients respond to lower doses of these U-100 insulins (usually 10–30 units). A1C

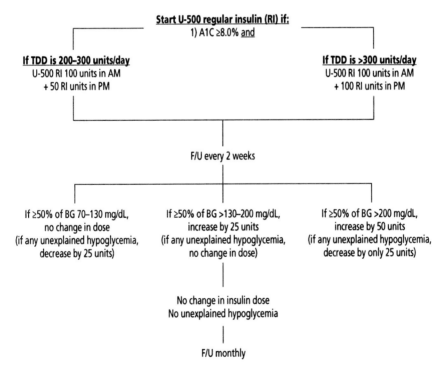

Figure 3.7. Flow diagram describing the initiation and dose adjustments of Humulin U-500 regular insulin. BG, blood glucose; F/U, follow-up; RI, regular insulin; TDD, total daily dose. Reprinted with permission from Ballani et al.[111]

levels can often be lowered to <7.5% and routinely to <8.0% with Humulin U-500 regular insulin.[110]

Single before-breakfast injection of NPH insulin

If a single morning injection is used, near-euglycemia is seldom achieved. This approach requires that the single morning injection of NPH insulin control both the before-supper glucose concentration and the following morning's value. The usual scenario is that as the morning NPH insulin dose is raised, the before-supper glucose concentrations become acceptable before the fasting values. As the NPH insulin dose is increased still further to lower the before-breakfast concentrations, late-afternoon hypoglycemia occurs, and the morning NPH insulin dose must be stabilized or decreased before target fasting levels are reached. At this point, evening NPH insulin must be introduced to improve control further (i.e., the patient is now on a self-mixed/split regimen, which should have been the initial approach).

There are three exceptions to this scenario. A few patients with type 2 diabetes who fail noninsulin medications have FPG values at target or very near target. Their elevated A1C levels are due to daytime hyperglycemia, most often manifested by high before-supper SMBG results. In that situation, before-breakfast NPH insulin is indicated, initially 10 units in lean patients and 16 units in overweight/obese patients. Eventually, as endogenous insulin secretion continues to decrease, evening NPH insulin often becomes necessary.

A second exception occurs in patients taking large doses of prednisone in the morning only. This steroid will cause daytime insulin resistance but its effect wanes overnight. In this case, many of these patients can be controlled on a single dose of NPH insulin before breakfast, although often short- or rapid-acting insulin is also necessary before breakfast and sometimes also before supper.

A third rare exception to the requirement of two injections of NPH insulin is the patient who has a delayed response to NPH insulin, i.e., the peak effect of a morning injection occurs overnight so that the next day's fasting glucose concentration is affected more than the before-supper value.[112,113] In this unusual situation, a single morning injection of NPH insulin is appropriate, with short- or rapid-acting insulin given preprandially as necessary. Interestingly, the pharmacodynamic response to short- and rapid-acting insulin remains normal. This result suggests that the reason for the delayed response involves a slowed release of insulin from the protamine in the NPH preparation rather than a general delay in the egress of insulin from the subcutaneous space into the circulation. Patients with a delayed response to NPH insulin are usually identified by recognizing that the FPG concentrations remain low as the evening NPH insulin dose in a self-mixed/split regimen continues to be reduced and remains normal or low, even when no evening NPH insulin is injected. These patients can be challenging to control. The FPG concentration reflects the action of the previous morning's NPH insulin. That dose is changed according to the pattern of FPG values. Preprandial short- or rapid-acting insulin is then necessary to control glucose concentrations during the day. Essentially, these patients are on a basal/bolus regimen with the basal insulin being the before-breakfast NPH insulin. Fortunately, this delayed response to NPH insulin does not occur often.

We recently followed a patient receiving Humulin U-500 regular insulin who also had a delayed response to this insulin preparation.[114] This patient casts doubt on the suggested mechanism described above that the cause of a delayed peak pattern to NPH insulin is a slower dissociation of insulin from the protamine because the U-500 insulin preparation does not contain protamine.

Intensified insulin regimens as initial therapy

As discussed previously, most patients with type 2 diabetes will transition to insulin therapy via either bedtime NPH or a basal insulin. A few patients newly diagnosed with type 2 diabetes with markedly elevated glucose concentrations will (unnecessarily) be initially treated with insulin, and the usual subsequent therapeutic activity is to decrease the doses and often to safely discontinue insulin by substituting noninsulin medication(s). Patients with type 1 diabetes who present in diabetic DKA will be discharged from the hospital on insulin. However, there are some patients who may benefit from an initial intensified insulin regimen, e.g., patients with type 1 diabetes diagnosed before DKA supervenes, patients with LADA failing control with noninsulin medications in whom it is felt that a more gradual approach with bedtime NPH or a basal insulin is inappropriate, and patients with type 2 diabetes with a long duration of diabetes poorly controlled on noninsulin medications. Initial doses of a self-mixed/split and basal/bolus regimens are presented in Table 3.13 for both overweight/obese and lean patients. As with other regimens, these initial doses are most often much less than eventually required to limit hypoglycemia, which may discourage patients from continuing with insulin therapy.

Table 3.13. Initial Insulin Doses for Intensified Regimens

Overweight and obese subjects			
Before breakfast	Before lunch	Before supper	Before bedtime
20 units NPH/4–6 units short- or rapid- acting insulin	–	10 units NPH/4–6 units short- or rapid-acting insulin	–
6–8 units short- or rapid-acting insulin	6–8 units short- or rapid-acting insulin	6–8 units short- or rapid-acting insulin	16 units NPH or basal insulin
Lean subjects			
Before breakfast	Before lunch	Before supper	Before bedtime
10 units NPH/2–4 units short- or rapid- acting insulin	–	6 units NPH/2–4 units short- or rapid-acting insulin	–
4 units short- or rapid-acting insulin	4 units short- or rapid-acting insulin	4 units short- or rapid-acting insulin	10 units NPH or basal insulin

REFERENCES

1. American Diabetes Association. Glycemic targets. *Diabetes Care* 2016;39(Suppl. 1):S39–S46

2. Holman RR. Assessing the potential for α-glucosidase inhibitors in prediabetic states. *Diabetes Res Clin Pract* 1998;40(Suppl.):S21–S25

3. Inzucchi SE, Bergenstal RM, Buse JB, et al. Management of hyperglycemia in type 2 diabetes, 2015: a patient-centered approach. Update to a position statement of the American Diabetes Association and the European Association for the Study of Diabetes. *Diabetes Care* 2015;38:140–149

4. Sherifali D, Nerenberg K, Pullenayegum E, et al. The effect of oral antidiabetic agents on A1C levels: a systematic review and meta-analysis. *Diabetes Care* 2010;33:1859–1864

5. Phung OJ, Scholle JM, Talwar M, Coleman CI. Effect of noninsulin antidiabetic drugs added to metformin therapy on glycemic control, weight gain, and hypoglycemia in type 2 diabetes. *JAMA* 2010;303:1410–1418

6. Gross JL, Kramer CK, Leitao CB, et al.; the Diabetes and Endocrinology Meta-analysis Group (DEMA). Effect of antihyperglycemic agents added to metformin and a sulfonylurea on glycemic control and weight gain in type 2 diabetes: a network meta-analysis. *Ann Intern Med* 2011;154:672–679

7. Bennett WL, Maruthur NM, Singh S, et al. Comparative effectiveness and safety of medications for type 2 diabetes: an update including new drugs and 2-drug combinations. *Ann Intern Med* 2011;154:602–613

8. Hsia SH, Navar M, Duran P, et al. Sitagliptin compared with thiazolidinediones as a third-line oral antihyperglycemic agent in type 2 diabetes mellitus. *Endocr Pract* 2011;17:691–698

9. Ferrannini E, Berk A, Hantel S, et al. Long-term safety and efficacy of empagliflozin, sitagliptin, and metformin. *Diabetes Care* 2013;36:4015–4021

10. Cefalu WT, Leiter LA, Yoon K-H, et al. Efficacy and safety of canagliflozin versus glimepiride in patients with type 2 diabetes inadequately controlled with metformin (CANATA-SU): 52 week results from a randomized, double-blind, phase 3 non-inferiority trial. *Lancet* 2013;382:941–950

11. Ridderstrale M, Andersen KR, Zeller C, et al.; EMPA-REG H2H-SU Trial Investigators. Comparison of empagliflozin and glimepiride as add-on to metformin in patients with type 2 diabetes: a 104 week randomized, active-controlled, double-blind, phase 3 trial. *Lancet Diabetes Endocrinol* 2014;2:691–700

12. Leiter LA, Yoon K-H, Arias P, et al. Canagliflozin provides durable glycemic improvements and body weight reduction over 104 weeks versus glimepiride in patients with type 2 diabetes on metformin: a randomized, double-blind, phase 3 study. *Diabetes Care* 2015;38:355–364

13. Schernthaner G, Gross JL, Rosenstock J, et al. Canagliflozin compared with sitagliptin for patients with type 2 diabetes who do not have adequate glycemic control with metformin plus sulfonylurea: a 52 week randomized trial. *Diabetes Care* 2013;36:2508–2515

14. Lavalle-Gonzalez FJ, Januszewicz A, Davidson J, et al. Efficacy and safety of canagliflozin compared with placebo and sitagliptin in patients with type 2 diabetes on background metformin monotherapy: a randomized trial. *Diabetologia* 2013;56:2582–2592

15. Lewin A, DeFronzo RA, Patel S, et al. Initial combination of empagliflozin and linagliptin in subjects with type 2 diabetes. *Diabetes Care* 2015;38:394–402

16. DeFronzo RA, Lewin A, Patel S, et al. Combination of empagliflozin and linagliptin as second-line therapy in subjects inadequately controlled on metformin. *Diabetes Care* 2015;38:384–393

17. Rosenstock J, Hansen L, Zee P, et al. Dual add-on therapy in type 2 diabetes poorly controlled with metformin monotherapy: a randomized double-blind trial of saxagliptin plus dapagliflozin addition versus single addition of saxagliptin or dapagliflozin to metformin. *Diabetes Care* 2015;38:376–383

18. American Diabetes Association. Approaches to glycemic treatment. *Diabetes Care* 2016;39(Suppl. 1):S52–S59

19. Peters AL, Davidson MB. Maximal dose glyburide therapy in markedly symptomatic patients with type 2 diabetes: a new use for an old friend. *J Clin Endocrinol Metab* 1996;81:2423–2427

20. Babu A, Mehta A, Guerrero P, et al. Safe and simple emergency department discharge therapy for patients with type 2 diabetes mellitus and severe hyperglycemia. *Endocr Pract* 2009;15:696–704

21. Amblee A, Lious D, Fogelfeld L. Combination of saxagliptin and metformin is effective as initial therapy in new-onset type 2 diabetes mellitus with severe hyperglycemia. *J Clin Endocrinol Metab* 2016;101:2528–2535

22. Kosaka K, Mizuno Y, Kuzuya T. Reproducibility of the oral glucose tolerance test and the rice-meal test in mild diabetics. *Diabetes* 1966;15:901–904

23. Ollerton RL, Playle R, Ahmed K, et al. Day-to-day variability of fasting plasma glucose in newly diagnosed type 2 diabetic subjects. *Diabetes Care* 1999;22:394–398

24. Garber AJ, Duncan TG, Goodman AM, et al. Efficacy of metformin in type II diabetes: results of a double-blind, placebo-controlled, dose-response trial. *Am J Med* 1997;102:491–497

25. Shaw JS, Wilmot RL, Kilpatrick ES. Establishing pragmatic estimated GFR thresholds to guide metformin prescribing. *Diabet Med* 2007;24:1160–1163

26. Inzucchi SE, Lipska KJ, Mayo H, et al. Metformin in patients with type 2 diabetes and kidney disease: a systemic review. *JAMA* 2014;312:2668–2675

27. Manual on Contrast Media v10.1: American College of Radiology. Available at http://www.acr.org/quality-safety/resources/contrast-manual. Accessed 10 October 2016

28. Salpeter SR, Greyber E, Pasternak GA, Salpeter EE. Risk of fatal and non-fatal lactic acidosis with metformin in type 2 diabetes mellitus. *Cochrane Database Syst Rev* 2010;1:CD002967

29. Bodmer M, Meier C, Kruhenbuhl S, et al. Metformin, sulfonylureas, or other antidiabetic drugs and the risk of lactic acidosis or hypoglycemia: a nested case-control analysis. *Diabetes Care* 2008;31;2086–2091

30. Billington EO, Grey A, Bolland MJ. Decreases in bone mineral density following treatment with thiazolinediones. *Diabetologia* 2015;58:2238–2246

31. Habib ZA, Havstad SL, Wells K, et al. Thiazolidinedione use and the longitudinal risk of fractures in patients with type 2 diabetes mellitus. *J Clin Endocrinol Metab* 2010;95:592–600

32. Lewis JD, Ferrara A, Peng T, et al. Risk of bladder cancer among diabetic patients treated with pioglitazone: report of a longitudinal cohort study. *Diabetes Care* 2011;34:916–922

33. Lewis JD, Habel LA, Quesenberry CP, et al. Pioglitazone use and risk of baldder cancer and other common cancers in persons with diabetes. *JAMA* 2015;314:265–277

34. Davidson MB. Pioglitazone (Actos) and bladder cancer: legal system triumphs over the evidence. *J Diabetes and Its Complications* 2016;30:981-985

35. Janci MM, Smith RC, Soule P. Polycystic ovarian syndrome: metformin or thiazolidinediones for cardiovascular risk reduction. *Diabetes Spectrum* 2012;25:229–237

36. Nissen SE, Wolski K. Effect of rosiglitazone on the risk of myocardial infarction and death from cardiovascular causes. *N Engl J Med* 2006;356:2457–2471

37. Home PD, Pocock SJ, Beck-Nielsen H, et al. Rosiglitazone Evaluated for Cardiovascular Outcomes in Oral Agent Combination Therapy for Type 2 Diabetes (RECORD): a multicentre, randomized, open-label trial. *Lancet* 2009;373:2125–2135

38. Kaplan K. FDA affirms safety of diabetes drug Avandia, lifts restrictions on use. http://www.latimes.com/science/sciencenow/la-sci-sn-avandia-fda-diabetes-drug-20131125-story.html. Accessed 10 March 2016

39. Mazzone T, Meyer PM, Feinstein SB, et al. Effect of pioglitazone compared with glimepiride on carotid intima-media thickness in type 2 diabetes: a randomized trial. *JAMA* 2006;296:2572–2581

40. Nissen SE, Nicholls SJ, Wolski K, et al.; PERISCOPE Investigators. Comparison of pioglitazone vs glimepiride on progression of coronary athero-

sclerosis in patients with type 2 diabetes: the PERISCOPE randomized controlled trial. *JAMA* 2008;299:1561–1573

41. Patel D, Walitt B, Lindsay J, Wilensky RL. Role of pioglitazone in the prevention of restenosis and need for revascularization after bare-metal stent implantation: a meta-analysis. *JACC Cardiovasc Interv* 2011;4:353–360

42. Dormandy JA, Charbonnel B, Eckland DJA, et al. Secondary prevention of macrovascular events in patients with type 1 diabetes in the PROactive Study (PROspective pioglitAzone Clinical Trial In macroVascular Events): a randomized controlled trial. *Lancet* 2005;366:1279–1289

43. Lincoff AM, Wolski K, Nicholls SJ, Nissen SE. Pioglitazone and risk of cardiovascular events in patient with type 2 diabetes mellitus: a meta-analysis of randomized trials. *JAMA* 2007;298:1180–1188

44. Erdmann E, Dormandy JA, Charbonnel B, on behalf of the PROactive Investigators. The effect of pioglitazone on recurrent myocardial infarction in 2,445 patients with type 2 diabetes and previous myocardial infarction. *J Am Coll Cardiol* 2007;49:1772–1780

45. Wilcox R, Bousser M-G, Betteridge J, et al.; PROactive Investigators. Effects of pioglitazone in patients with type 2 diabetes with or without previous stroke: results from PROactive (PROspective pioglitAzone Clinical Trial macroVascular Events 04). *Stroke* 2007;38:865–873

46. Dormandy JA, Betteridge DJ, Schernthaner G, et al.; PROactive Investigators. Impact of peripheral arterial disease in patients with diabetes-results from PROactive (PROactive 11). *Atherosclerosis* 2009;202:272–281

47. Althouse AD, Abbott JD, Sutton-Tyrrell K, et al.; BARI 2D Study Group. Favorable effects of insulin sensitizers pertinent to peripheral arterial disease in type 2 diabetes: results from the Bypass Angioplasty Revascularization Investigation 2 Diabetes (BARI 2D) trial. *Diabetes Care* 2014;37:1346–1352

48. Suarez EA, Koro CE, Christian JB, et al. Incretin-mimetic therapies and pancreatic disease: a review of observational data. *Curr Med Res Opin* 2014;30:2471–2481

49. Gokhale M, Buse JB, Gray LB, et al. Dipeptidyl-peptidase-4 inhibitors and pancreatic cancers: a cohort study. *Diabetes Metab Obes* 2014;16:1247–1256

50. Knapen LM, van Dalem J, Keulemans YC, et al. Use of incretin agents and risk of pancreatic cancer: a population-based cohort study. *Diabetes Obes Metab* 2016;18:258–265

51. Azoulay L, Filion K, Platt RW, et al.; Canadian Network for Observational Drug Effect Studies (CNODES) Investigators. Incretin based drugs and the risk of pancreatic cancer: international multicenter cohort study. *BMJ* 2016;352:i581 doi: 10.1136

52. Marso SP, Daniels GH, Brown-Frandsen K, et al. Liraglutide and cardiovascular outcomes in type 2 diabetes. *N Engl J Med* 2016;375:311–322

53. Marso SP, Bain SC, Consoli A, et al. Semaglutide and cardiovascular outcomes in patients with type 2 diabetes. N Engl J Med. 2016;375:1834-1844

54. Pfeiffer MA, Claggett B, Diaz R, et al. Lixisenatide in patients with type 2 diabetes and acute coronary syndrome. *N Engl J Med* 2015;373:2247–2257

55. Karagiannis T, Paschos P, Paletas K, et al. Dipeptidyl peptidase-4 inhibitors for treatment of type 2 diabetes mellitus in the clinical setting: systematic review and meta-analysis. *BMJ* 2012;344:e1369 doi: 10.1136bmj.e1369

56. Scirica BM, Bhatt DL, Braunwald E, et al. Saxagliptin and cardiovascular outcomes in patients with type 2 diabetes mellitus. *N Engl J Med* 2013;369:1317–1326

57. Yu OHY, Filion KB, Azoulay L, et al. Incretin-based drugs and the risk of congestive heart failure. *Diabetes Care* 2015;38:277–284

58. Fu AZ, Johnston SS, Ghannom A, et al. Association between hospitalization for heart failure and dipeptidyl peptidase-4 inhibitors in patients with type 2 diabetes: an observational study. *Diabetes Care* 2016;39:726–734

59. Hasan FM, Alsahi M, Gerich JE. SGLT2 inhibitors in the treatment of type 2 diabetes. *Diabetes Res Clin Pract* 2014;104:297–322

60. Erondu N, Desai M, Meininger G. Diabetic ketoacidosis and related events in the canagliflozin type 2 diabetes clinical program. *Diabetes Care* 2015;38:1680–1686

61. Henry RR, Thakkar P, Tong C, et al. Efficacy and safety of canagliflozin, a sodium–glucose cotransporter 2 inhibitor, as add-on to insulin in patients with type 1 diabetes. *Diabetes Care* 2015;38:2258–2265

62. FDA Drug Safety Communication: FDA revises labels of SGLT2 inhibitors for diabetes to include warnings about too much acid in the blood and serious urinary tract infections. Available at www.fda.gov/Drugs/DrugSafety/ucm475463.htm. Accessed 25 December 2016

63. FDA Warns Invokana May Increase Risk of Bone Fractures. Available at https://www.drugwatch.com. Accessed 25 December 2016

64. Zinman B, Wanner C, Lachin JM, et al. Empagliflozin, cardiovascular outcomes, and mortality in type 2 diabetes. *N Engl J Med* 2015;373:2117–2128

65. Western Health, Acarbose. Available at westernhealth.nl.ca/uploads/Diabetes/Acarbose.pdf. Accessed 25 December 2016

66. DeFronzo RA. Bromocriptine: a sympatholytic, D2-dopamine agonist for the treatment of type 2 diabetes. *Diabetes Care* 2011;34:789–794; erratum *Diabetes Care* 2011;34:1442

67. Gaziano JM, Cincotta AH, O'Connor CM, et al. Randomized clinical trial of quick-release bromocriptine among patients with type2 diabetes on overall safety and cardiovascular outcomes. *Diabetes Care* 2010;33:1503–1508

68. Karter AJ, Ackerson LM, Darbinian JA, et al. Self-monitoring of blood glucose levels and glycemic control: the Northern California Kaiser Permanente Diabetes Registry. *Am J Med* 2001;111:1–9

69. Schutt SM, Kern W, Krause U, et al.; DPV Initiative. Is the frequency of self-monitoring of blood glucose related to long-term metabolic control? Multicenter analysis including 24,500 patients from 191 centers in Germany and Austria. *Exp Clin Endocrinol Diabetes* 2006;114:384–388

70. Davidson MB. Evaluation of self monitoring of blood glucose in non-insulin-treated diabetic patients by randomized controlled trials: little bang for the buck. *Rev Recent Clin Trials* 2010;5:138–142

71. Farmer AJ, Perera R, Ward A, et al. Meta-analysis of individual patient data in randomized trials of self-monitoring of blood glucose in people with non-insulin treated type 2 diabetes. *BMJ* 2012;344:e486 doi:10.1136bmj.e486

72. Malanda UL, Welschen LM, Riphagen II, et al. Self-monitoring of blood glucose in patients with type 2 diabetes mellitus who are not using insulin. *Cochrane Database Syst Rev* 2012;1:CD005060

73. Duran A, Martin P, Runkle I, et al. Benefits of self-monitoring blood glucose in the management of new-onset type 2 diabetes mellitus: the St Carlos Study, a prospective randomized clinic-based interventional study with parallel groups. *J Diabetes* 2010;2:203–211

74. Polonsky WH, Fisher L, Schikman CH, et al. Structured self-monitoring of blood glucose significantly reduces A1C levels in poorly controlled, noninsulin-treated type 2 diabetes. *Diabetes Care* 2011;34:262–267

75. Pimazoni-Netto A, Rodbard D, Zanella MT, on behalf of the Diabetes Education and Control Group. Rapid improvement of glycemic control in type 2 diabetes using weekly intensive multifactorial interventions: structured glucose monitoring, patient education, and adjustment of therapy: a randomized controlled trial. *Diabetes Tech Therap* 2011;13:997–1004

76. Franciosi M, Lucisano G, Pellegrini F, et al. ROSES: role of self-monitoring of blood glucose and intensive education in patients with type 2 diabetes not receiving insulin: a pilot randomized clinical trial. *Diabet Med* 2011;28:789–796

77. Davidson MB: How our current medical care system fails people with diabetes: lack of timely, appropriate clinical decisions. *Diabetes Care* 2009;32:370–372

78. Akbaraly TN, Tabak AG, Shipley MJ, et al. Little change in diet after onset of type 2 diabetes, metabolic syndrome, and obesity in middle-aged adults: 11-year follow up study. *Diabetes Care* 2016;39:e29–e30

79. Davidson MB. Self monitoring of blood glucose in type 2 diabetic patients not receiving insulin: a waste of money. *Diabetes Care* 2005;28:1531–1533

80. Davidson MB, Castellanos M, Duran P, Karlan V. Effective diabetes care by a registered nurse following treatment algorithms in a minority population. *Am J Manag Care* 2006;12:226–232

81. American Diabetes Association. Diabetes and driving. *Diabetes Care* 2014;37(Suppl. 1):S97–S103

82. Davidson MB: Insulin analogues: is there a compelling case to use them? No! *Diabetes Care* 2014;37:1771–1774

83. Vora J, Cariou B, Evans M, et al. Clinical use of insulin degludec. *Diabetes Res Clin Pract* 2015;109:19–31

84. Davies M, Sasaki T, Gross JL, et al. Comparison of insulin degludec with insulin detemir in type 1 diabetes: a 1-year treat-to-target trial. *Diabetes Obes Metab* 2016;18:96–99

85. Ziel FH, Davidson MB, Harris MD, Rosenberg CS. The variability in the action of regular insulin is more dependent on changes in tissue sensitivity than on insulin absorption. *Diabet Med* 1988;5:662–666

86. Heinemann L. Variability of insulin absorption and insulin action. *Diabetes Tech Ther* 2002;4:673–682

87. Muller N, Frank T, Kloos C, et al. Randomized crossover study to examine the necessity of an injection-to-meal interval in patients with type 2 diabetes mellitus and human insulin. *Diabetes Care* 2013;36:1865–1869

88. Seaquist ER, Anderson J, Childs B, et al. Hypoglycemia and diabetes: a report of a work group of the American Diabetes Association and the Endocrine Society. *Diabetes Care* 2013;36:1384–1395

89. Hamwi GJ. Therapy: changing dietary concepts. In *Diabetes Mellitus: Diagnosis and Treatment*. Vol. 1. Danowski TS, Ed. New York, American Diabetes Association, 1964, p. 73–78

90. Yki-Jarvinen H, Kauppila M, Kujansuu E, et al. Comparison of insulin regimens in patients with non-insulin-dependent diabetes mellitus. *N Engl J Med* 1992;327:1426–1433

91. Wolffenbuttal BH, Sets JP, Rondas-Colbers GJ, et al. Comparison of different regimens in elderly patients with NIDDM. *Diabetes Care* 1996;19:1326–1332

92. Yki-Jarvinen H, Ryysy L, Kauppila M, et al. Effect of obesity on the response to insulin therapy in noninsulin-dependent diabetes mellitus. *J Clin Endocrinol Metab* 1997;82:4037–4043

93. Yki-Jarvinen H, Ryysy L, Nikkila K, et al. Comparison of bedtime insulin in patients with type 2 diabetes mellitus: a randomized, controlled trial. *Ann Intern Med* 1999;130:389–396

94. Cusi K, Cunningham GR, Comstock JP. Safety and efficacy of normalizing fasting glucose with bedtime NPH insulin alone in NIDDM. *Diabetes Care* 1995;18;843–851

95. Tahara Y, Shima K. The response of GHb to stepwise plasma glucose change over time in diabetic patients. *Diabetes Care* 1993;16:1313–1314

96. Racah, Bretzel RG, Owens D, Riddle M. When basal insulin therapy in type 2 diabetes mellitus is not enough: what next? *Diabetes Metab Res Rev* 2007;23:257–264

97. Owens DR, Luzio SD, Sert-Langeron C, Riddle MC. Effects of initiation and titration of a single pre-prandial dose of insulin glulisine while continuing titrated insulin glargine in type 2 diabetes: a 6 month "proof of concept" study. *Diabetes Obes Metab* 2011;13:1020–1027

98. Davidson MB, Raskin P, Tanenberg RJ, et al. A stepwise approach to insulin therapy in patients with type 2 diabetes and basal insulin treatment failure. *Endocr Pract* 2011;17:395–403

99. Fulcher G, Roberts A, Sinha A, Proietta J. What happens when patients require intensification from basal insulin? A retrospective audit of clinical practice for the treatment of type 2 diabetes from four Australian centres. *Diabetes Res Clin Pract* 2015;108:405–413

100. Rodbard H, Visco VE, Andersen H, Hiort LC, Shu DHW. Treatment intensification with stepwise addition of prandial insulin aspart boluses compared with full basal-bolus therapy (FullSTEP Study): a randomized, treat-to-target clinical trial. *Lancet Diabetes Endocrinol* 2014;2:30–37

101. Monnier L, Colette C, Dunseath GJ, Owens DR. The loss of postprandial glycemic control precedes stepwise deterioration of fasting with worsening diabetes. *Diabetes Care* 2007;30:263–269

102. Bonomo K, DeSalve A, Fiova E, et al. Evaluation of a simple policy for pre- and post-prandial blood glucose self-monitoring in people with type 2 diabetes not on insulin. *Diabetes Res Clin Pract* 2010;87:246–251

103. Davidson MB. The self-mixed/split insulin regimen: a serious omission in the ADA/EASD Position Statement. *Diabetes Care* 2014;37:3–4

104. Reeves ML, Seigler DE, Ryan EA, Skyler JS. Glycemic control in insulin-dependent diabetes mellitus: comparison of outpatient intensified conventional therapy with continuous subcutaneous insulin infusion. *Am J Med* 1982;72:673–680

105. Umpierrez GE, Hor T, Smiley D, et al. Comparison of inpatient insulin regimens with detemir plus aspart *versus* neutral protamne Hagedorn plus regular in medical patients with type 2 diabetes. *J Clin Endocrinol Metab* 2009;94:564–569

106. Kulkarni K. Carbohydrate counting for pump therapy. In *A Core Curriculum for Diabetes Education: Diabetes Management Therapies*. 5th ed. Franz MJ, Ed. American Association of Diabetes Educators, 2003, p. 265–276

107. Bergenstal RM, Johnson M, Powers MA, et al. Adjust to target in type 2 diabetes: comparison of a simple algorithm with carbohydrate counting for adjustment of mealtime insulin glulisine. *Diabetes Care* 2008;31:1305–1310

108. Scherthaner-RA, Wein W, Shnawa N, et al. Preprandial vs. postprandial insulin: a comparative crossover trial in patients with Type 1 diabetes. *Diabet Med* 2004;21:279–284

109. Binder C. Absorption of injected insulin: a clinical-pharmacological study. *Acta Pharmacol Toxicol* 1969;27(Suppl. 2):11–87

110. Davidson MB, Navar MD, Echeverry D, Duran P. U-500 regular insulin: clinical experience and pharmacokinetics in obese, severely insulin-resistant type 2 diabetic patients. *Diabetes Care* 2010;33:281–283

111. Ballani P, Tran MT, Navar MD, Davidson MB. Clinical experience with U-500 regular insulin in obese, markedly insulin resistant type 2 diabetic patients. *Diabetes Care* 2006;29:2504–2505; errata *Diabetes Care* 2007;30:455

112. Davidson MB. Delayed response to NPH insulin. *Diab Res Clin Pract* 2004;64:229

113. Davidson MB. Delayed response to NPH insulin. In *Diabetes Case Files: Real Problems, Practical Solutions*. Draznin B, Ed. Alexandria, VA, American Diabetes Association, 2014, p. 267–270

114. Davidson MB. Delayed response to U-500 regular insulin. *Clinical Diabetes*. In press.

115. Kernan WN, Viscoli CM, Furie KL, et al.; IRIS Trial Investigators. Pioglitazone after ischemic stroke or transient ischemic attack. *N Engl J Med* 2016;374:1321–1331

116. Chiasson J-L, Josse RG, Gomis R, et al.; STOP-NIDDM Trial Research Group. Acarbose for prevention of type 2 diabetes mellitus: the STOP-NIDDM randomized trial. *Lancet* 2002;359:2072–2077

117. UK Prospective Diabetes Study (UKPDS) Group. Intensive blood glucose control with sulphonylureas or insulin compared with conventional treatment and risk of complications in patients with type 2 diabetes (UKPDS 33). *Lancet* 1998;352:837–853

118. UK Prospective Diabetes Study (UKPDS) Group. Effect of intensive blood control with metformin on complications in overweight patients with type 1 diabetes (UKPDS 34). *Lancet* 1998;352:854–865

Chapter 4
Dyslipidemia

HYPERCHOLESTEROLEMIA AND ASCVD

Several population-based prospective cohort studies have shown that the risk of atherosclerotic cardiovascular disease (ASCVD) death and other ASCVD events in individuals with diabetes is similar to that of nondiabetic individuals who already had a history of myocardial infarction,[1-3] an observation that has prompted the designation of diabetes as a "coronary disease equivalent." As previously discussed in Chapter 1, there is now a large body of literature showing that LDL cholesterol lowering with HMG-CoA reductase inhibitors (statins) can effectively reduce ASCVD events and prolong survival.[4-6] For patients with diabetes, studies like the Collaborative Atorvastatin Diabetes Study (CARDS)[7] as well as subgroup analyses of the diabetes patients in several major statin intervention trials[8-16] and a meta-analysis of diabetes patients from major statin trials[17] all showed that the relative risk reduction for ASCVD events in individuals with diabetes is similar to that for nondiabetic individuals. However, because individuals with diabetes have a higher background absolute risk of ASCVD events than comparable nondiabetic individuals, this means that individuals with diabetes actually benefit from a larger absolute risk reduction[17] (i.e., a higher actual number of ASCVD events prevented, such that the percent reduction is similar).

For the general population, currently accepted treatment guidelines to lower LDL cholesterol fall along two different strategies. The guidelines of the National Cholesterol Education Program's Third Adult Treatment Panel (ATP-III) advocate treating LDL cholesterol down below an absolute LDL cholesterol goal level based on the patient's risk profile, with a lower goal being recommended for higher-risk individuals. For diabetes patients, ATP-III recommends that LDL cholesterol be reduced to <100 mg/dL, and for diabetes patients who additionally have a history of ASCVD (e.g., previous myocardial infarction, stroke, or other clinically significant atherosclerotic disease), LDL cholesterol should be reduced to <70 mg/dL.[18,19] In contrast, the 2013 guidelines of the American College of Cardiology and American Heart Association (ACC/AHA) more simply advocate the use of statin dosages of sufficient LDL cholesterol–lowering effect, independent of the absolute LDL cholesterol levels achieved, with a greater relative reduction from baseline being recommended for higher-risk individuals. For diabetes patients age ≥40 years, use of a "moderate-intensity" or "high-intensity" statin dosage that can achieve a lowering of LDL cholesterol by 30–50% or ≥50% from baseline, respectively, is recommended.[20] At present, there is disagreement as to which strategy may be the best clinical approach, and no comparative scientific

DOI: 10.2337/9781580406017.04

evidence exists to support an advantage of either approach for ASCVD outcomes. The ACC/AHA guidelines were developed based solely on a strict interpretation of evidence from high-quality randomized controlled trials that used only fixed doses of statins, either in comparison to placebo or as a comparison between different fixed doses, so they are a faithful interpretation of the available scientific evidence. However, the ATP-III guidelines were developed based on the more traditional principle of "the lower the cholesterol, the better," a concept that has become familiar to many clinicians (and perhaps patients, too) and that is supported by extensive population-based observational evidence.[21-23] However, no randomized controlled trials have ever addressed that specific hypothesis. Even now, large cross-sectional surveys both in the U.S. and internationally still show that, for a substantial proportion of the population, cholesterol levels are not optimally controlled below the ATP-III–recommended targets,[24,25] so there is concern among some clinicians that the ACC/AHA guidelines do not facilitate the more aggressive use of statins that many feel is necessary. However, the strong evidence basis underlying the ACC/AHA guidelines is undeniable.

PRINCIPLES OF HYPERCHOLESTEROLEMIA TREATMENT

The American Diabetes Association (ADA) recommends that a fasting lipid profile be obtained on all patients with diabetes at the time of initial diagnosis or at the patient's initial medical evaluation and then at least every 5 years thereafter (or more frequently, based on individual clinical judgment).[26] Routine lipid profiles do not directly measure LDL cholesterol but instead derive the level based on measurements of total cholesterol, HDL cholesterol, and triglycerides (TGs) and then calculate LDL cholesterol level using the classic Friedewald equation:

$$\text{LDL cholesterol} = \text{total cholesterol} - \text{HDL cholesterol} - [\text{TGs}/5]$$

This equation is not valid for any TG level ≥400 mg/dL, so for a patient who has not adequately fasted or has an underlying TG disorder and has this degree of hypertriglyceridemia, LDL cholesterol cannot be reliably calculated. If an adequate fast fails to reduce TGs <400 mg/dL, direct LDL assays (if available) can specifically measure the LDL cholesterol, but aside from entailing additional expense (so they should not be performed routinely), the high TG level can still cause these assays to underestimate LDL cholesterol as well as ASCVD risk classification in some patients.[27] Nevertheless, in such cases, they do provide the clinician with an LDL cholesterol level where there otherwise would be no reliable value at all. The specific management of hypertriglyceridemia will be discussed later in this chapter.

Medical nutrition therapy and lifestyle management should be taught to all patients with diabetes.[26] ATP-III recommends dietary and lifestyle management as a first-line intervention for any patient whose LDL cholesterol is above goal[18]; ACC/AHA also emphasizes lifestyle modification as a foundation of ASCVD prevention at all stages of statin therapy.[20] For cholesterol lowering, emphasis should be placed on aggressive reduction of dietary saturated and *trans* fats (i.e., not necessarily all dietary fat unless total calories are also a concern), as well as dietary cholesterol. Intake of dietary viscous fiber (e.g., contained in legumes, oats, citrus), omega-3 marine fish oils (ideally by eating two to three servings of fatty fish per week), and plant sterols/stanols should be encouraged, along with increased physical activity. For overweight or obese individuals, control of total calories also remains important.[26]

The ADA recently adapted its lipid management recommendations to largely follow the ACC/AHA guidelines.[26] Specifically, for patients with type 2 diabetes between the ages of 40 and 75 years (the age-group for whom evidence supports a benefit with statins), a statin of at least moderate-intensity should be used together with appropriate lifestyle modifications; for those with one or more additional ASCVD risk factors or a history of any overt ASCVD, a high-intensity statin is recommended (Tables 4.1 and 4.2). For diabetes patients over age 75 years, the evidence supporting a benefit of statins is weaker, but the same recommendations apply, along with greater attention to the risks associated with statin use and titration of high-intensity doses down to moderate-intensity doses when statin tolerability or drug interactions are a concern. Similarly, evidence for patients under age 40 years or patients with type 1 diabetes is also substantially weaker, but patients with a history of ASCVD should still be treated with a high-intensity statin, and patients with additional ASCVD risk factors should still be treated with a moderate- or high-intensity statin. Statin dosages that correspond to moderate or high intensity are shown in Table 4.2; statin dosages lower than these (i.e., "low intensity") generally do not produce ≥30% lowering of LDL cholesterol and are usually insufficient as long-term therapy.

Table 4.1. ADA Recommendations for Statin and Combination Treatment[26]

Age-group (years)	Risk factors	Recommended statin intensity*
<40	None	None
	ASCVD risk factor(s)**	Moderate or high
	ASCVD	High
40–75	None	Moderate
	ASCVD risk factor(s)**	High
	ASCVD	High
	ACS and LDL cholesterol >50 mg/dL in patients intolerant to high-dose statins	Moderate + ezetimibe
>75	None	Moderate
	ASCVD risk factor(s)**	Moderate or high
	ASCVD	High
	ACS and LDL cholesterol >50 mg/dL in patients intolerant to high-dose statins	Moderate + ezetimibe

*In addition to lifestyle therapy. **ASCVD risk factors include LDL cholesterol ≥100 mg/dL, high blood pressure, smoking, overweight or obesity, and family history of premature ASCVD. ACS, acute coronary syndrome.

Table 4.2. High-Intensity and Moderate-Intensity Statin Therapy (Once-Daily Doses)[26]

High-intensity statin therapy	Moderate-intensity statin therapy
LDL cholesterol lowering ≥50%	LDL cholesterol lowering 30% to <50%
Atorvastatin 40–80 mg Rosuvastatin 20–40 mg	Atorvastatin 10–20 mg Rosuvastatin 5–10 mg Simvastatin 20–40 mg Pravastatin 40–80 mg Lovastatin 40 mg Fluvastatin XL 80 mg Pitavastatin 2–4 mg

At out institution, because of formulary restrictions on the available statins, we opt for atorvastatin as a first-line choice at a starting dose of 10 mg daily (representing moderate intensity) or 40 mg daily (representing high intensity) (Table 4.3); in other settings, the equivalent doses of rosuvastatin may also be used. Our treatment approach begins in a manner analogous to the ADA fixed-dose statin recommendations. However, to maximize the benefits of statins, we additionally pursue the LDL cholesterol goals advocated by ATP-III (i.e., <100 mg/dL, or <70 mg/dL for patients with overt ASCVD) by doubling the respective doses if the starting doses still do not meet these absolute LDL cholesterol goals.

Individual patients may respond very differently to any given statin.[28] In general, lipid profiles should be reassessed monthly and statin treatment fur-

Table 4.3. Suggested Treatment Recommendations

Age-group (years)	Risk factors	Recommended starting statin dose
<40	None	None
	Risk factor(s)*	Atorvastatin 10 mg q.d./rosuvastatin 5 mg q.d.
	Overt ASCVD	Atorvastatin 40 mg q.d./rosuvastatin 20 mg q.d.
40–75	None	Atorvastatin 10 mg q.d./rosuvastatin 5 mg q.d.
	Risk factor(s) *	Atorvastatin 40 mg q.d./rosuvastatin 20 mg q.d.
	Overt ASCVD	Atorvastatin 40 mg q.d./rosuvastatin 20 mg q.d.
>75	None	Atorvastatin 10 mg q.d./rosuvastatin 5 mg q.d.
	Risk factor(s) *	Atorvastatin 10 mg q.d./rosuvastatin 5 mg q.d.
	Overt ASCVD	Atorvastatin 40 mg q.d./rosuvastatin 20 mg q.d.

*Risk factors include LDL cholesterol ≥100 mg/dL, hypertension (or use of anti-hypertension agents), smoking, and overweight or obesity (defined as BMI ≥27.0 or weight ≥120% of desirable body weight, as determined by methods such as that shown in Table 2.1).

ther intensified (i.e., doubled, at least until the maximum dose is reached) until the LDL cholesterol goal has been met. All statins are generally well tolerated (see Table 4.4). Aside from differences in LDL cholesterol–lowering efficacy, the ideal choice of a statin should also take into consideration the potential for drug interactions through the CYP3A4 system (e.g., macrolide antibiotics, imidazole antifungals, HIV protease inhibitors; pravastatin avoids the CYP system altogether and may interact less), other comorbid conditions that may increase toxicity (e.g., hypothyroidism, hepatic dysfunction, congenital myopathies), and the presence of renal insufficiency (e.g., the lower dose limits in Table 4.4 should be observed, with atorvastatin being the least dependent on renal clearance, making it a better choice for patients with renal insufficiency).[29] Elevations of liver transaminases occur uncommonly; regular monitoring of alanine aminotransferase (ALT) levels are generally not necessary unless there is underlying liver pathology (e.g., alcoholic cirrhosis, viral hepatitis). If the ALT progressively rises to greater than three times the upper limit of the normal (ULN) range, statin discontinuation will still allow eventual normalization of ALT. Myositis occurs even less commonly; regular surveillance of creatine phosphokinase (CK) levels is not necessary; it only needs to be measured if the patient complains of new onset or worsening of generalized myalgias. If the CK progressively rises to greater than 10 times the ULN, statin discontinuation will still allow eventual normalization of CK and myositis without long-term sequelae; however, if left untreated, rhabdomyolysis and progression to renal failure can occur. Complaints of myalgia occurring in the face of a normal CK level also pose a clinical challenge and usually require a trial of one or more alternate statins until a tolerable choice can be found. Lowering the dose or alternate-day dosing may also alleviate the discomfort, but the likelihood that LDL cholesterol goals can be achieved or sustained is substantially lower. Statins are also absolutely contraindicated during pregnancy and lactation.

If the goal has not been met at a maximum statin dose (or if the patient is intolerant to further dose increases or alternate statins of equal or greater intensity), combination therapy with the addition of ezetimibe is supported by the findings of the Improved Reduction of Outcomes: Vytorin Efficacy International Trial (IMPROVE-IT)[30] to further reduce adverse ASCVD events (a strategy that is also recognized by the ADA recommendations, as shown in Table 4.1). It should be noted that this is so far the only clinical trial evidence of sufficient quality to support an ASCVD benefit of a non-statin agent when added to background statin therapy. Other agents that principally lower LDL cholesterol (Table 4.4) also provide additive LDL cholesterol lowering when added to statins, but these medication classes are not yet supported by any clinical evidence of additive ASCVD event reduction. Bile acid sequestrants effectively lower LDL cholesterol[31] and can reduce ASCVD events when used as monotherapy,[32] but they can also increase TG levels (which can be mitigated somewhat by the concurrent statin). Their mode of action in the intestinal lumen often leads to bloating and constipation, and their binding action can interfere with the absorption of other concurrent medications if proper separation of dosing intervals is not followed. All of these cautions are less pronounced with colesevelam, a hydrogel tablet preparation, unlike colestipol and

Table 4.4. Currently Available Lipid-Lowering Agents in the U.S.

Generic name	Brand name(s)	Recommended starting dose[a]	Recommended dose increment	Maximum dose	Cautions
Statins					
Atorvastatin	Lipitor	≥10 mg q.d.[b]	Doubling	80 mg q.d.[b]	Myalgias/myositis ALT elevations (rare) Potential drug interactions
Rosuvastatin	Crestor	≥5 mg q.d.[b,c]	Doubling	40 mg q.d.[b,c]	
Simvastatin	Zocor	20 mg q.h.s.[d]	Doubling	40 mg q.h.s.	
Pravastatin	Pravachol	40 mg q.h.s.[e]	Doubling	80 mg q.h.s.	
Lovastatin	Mevacor	40 mg q.h.s.[f]	Doubling	80 mg q.h.s.[f]	
	Altoprev	40 mg q.h.s.[f]	Up to maximum	60 mg q.h.s.[f]	
Fluvastatin	Lescol	40 mg b.i.d.[g]	N/A	80 mg q.h.s.[g] or 40 mg b.i.d.[g]	
	Lescol XL	80 mg q.d.[g]	N/A	80 mg q.d.[g]	
Pitavastatin	Livalo	2 mg q.d.[b,h]	Doubling	4 mg q.d.[b,h]	
Cholesterol absorption inhibitor					
Ezetimibe	Zetia	10 mg q.d.	NA	10 mg q.d.	Upper respiratory symptoms Diarrhea Myalgias (uncommon if monotherapy)

Bile acid sequestrants				
Cholestyramine	Questran Questran Light Prevalite	4 g q.d. or b.i.d.* (4 g per packet/ scoop)	Additional 4 g	24 g daily* (q.d. to t.i.d.)	Constipation/gastrointestinal discomfort Hypertriglyceridemia Potential interference with drug absorption (side effects less pronounced with colesevelam)
Colestipol	Colestid	2 g q.d. or b.i.d.* (1 g per tablet) (Also available as 5 g per packet/scoop)	Additional 2–4 g	16 g daily* (q.d. to q.i.d.)	
Colesevelam	Welchol	3.75 g q.d. or 1.875 g b.i.d.* (0.625 g per tablet)	NA	3.75 g q.d. or 1.875 g b.i.d.*	
PCSK9 inhibitors					
Alirocumab	Praluent	75 mg s.c. every 2 weeks	Doubling	150 mg s.c. every 2 weeks	Injection site reactions Flu-like symptoms Myalgias/myositis (uncommon)
Evolocumab	Repatha	140 mg s.c. every 2 weeks or 420 mg s.c. every month	NA	140 mg s.c. every 2 weeks or 420 mg s.c. every month	

(continued on page 108)

Table 4.4. Currently Available Lipid-Lowering Agents in the U.S. *(continued)*

Generic name	Brand name(s)	Recommended starting dose[a]	Recommended dose increment	Maximum dose	Cautions
Fibrates[i]					
Gemfibrozil	Lopid	600 mg b.i.d.*	NA	600 mg b.i.d.*	Dyspepsia Myalgias/myositis ALT elevations Cholelithiasis
Fenofibrate	Fenoglide	40 mg q.d.*	Additional 40 mg	120 mg q.d.*	
	Lipofen	50 mg q.d.*	Additional 50 mg	150 mg q.d.*	
	Lofibra tablets	54 mg q.d.*	Additional 54 mg	160 mg q.d.*	
	Tricor	48 mg q.d.*	Additional 48 mg	145 mg q.d.*	
	Triglide	160 mg q.d.*	N/A	160 mg q.d.*	
Micronized fenofibrate[j]	Antara	30 mg q.d.*	Additional 30 mg	90 mg q.d.*	
	Lofibra capsules	67 mg q.d.*	Additional 67 mg	200 mg q.d.*	
Fenofibric acid[j]	Fibricor	35 mg q.d.	Additional 35 mg	105 mg q.d.	
	Trilipix	45 mg q.d.	Additional 45 mg	135 mg q.d.	
Nicotinic acid					
Niacin (immediate-release)	Niacor	250 mg* q.h.s.[k]	Additional 250 mg every 4–7 days up to 2,000 mg per day, then additional 250–500 mg every 2–4 weeks[k]	6,000 mg* daily (b.i.d. or t.i.d.)[k]	Flushing/pruritis ALT elevations Hyperuricemia Hyperglycemia Dyspepsia
Extended-release niacin	Niaspan Slo-Niacin	500 mg q.h.s.	Additional 500 mg	2,000 mg q.h.s.	

Omega-3 fatty acids[l]					
Omega-3 acid ethyl esters	Lovaza	2 g b.i.d. or 4 g q.d.* (465 mg EPA + 375 mg DHA per 1-g capsule)	NA	4 g daily* (q.d. or b.i.d.)	None
Icosapent ethyl	Vascepa	2 g b.i.d.* (EPA only)	NA	2 g b.i.d.*	
Other classes (restricted prescribing)[m]					
Lomitapide	Juxtapid	5 mg q.d.	Doubling	60 mg q.d.	Diarrhea / ALT elevations / Hepatic steatosis / Potential drug interactions
Mipomersen	Kynamro	200 mg s.c. every week	NA	200 mg s.c. every week	Injection site reactions / Flu-like symptoms / ALT elevations / Hepatic steatosis
Combination agents					
Ezetimibe/simvastatin	Vytorin	10 mg/20 mg q.h.s.	Doubling of simvastatin	10 mg/40 mg q.h.s.	Observe cautions of each individual agent

aBased on FDA-approved labeling, except for statins, which are based on the dose that achieves on average the minimum effective LDL cholesterol lowering (≥30% from baseline), but the response of an individual patient may vary. bCan be taken at any time of the day because of its long duration of action. cIn patients with severe renal insufficiency (creatinine clearance <30 mL/min): start at 5 mg q.d. and maximum dose 10 mg q.d. dStart at 5 mg q.h.s. eStart at 10 mg q.h.s. fUse caution if dose >20 mg/day. gUse has not been defined. hStart at 1 mg q.d. and maximum dose 2 mg q.d. even if creatinine clearance is 30–59 mL/min. iAll fibrate agents should be started at the lowest dose in patients with mild or moderate renal impairment and are contraindicated in patients with severe renal insufficiency (creatinine clearance <30 mL/min). jFenofibrate, micronized fenofibrate, and fenofibric acid differ based on bioavailability, but can be used interchangeably; fenofibrate is a pro-drug of fenofibric acid, which does not need to be taken with food. kSeveral different dose titration schemes exist for immediate-release niacin to improve the tolerability of side effects; individualized clinical judgment should be used. q.h.s. administration of the initial dose is intended to make the initial flushing less perceptible, but an initial daytime dose may also be considered; all daytime doses should ideally be administered with food to improve tolerability. In general, dose increments should not exceed 500 mg, increments should occur no faster than every 4–7 days, and any single dose ≥1,500 mg should be split up (b.i.d. or t.i.d.) and should not exceed 2,000 mg. An adequate therapeutic effect is usually seen at total daily doses ≥2,500 mg. lPrescription formulations of omega-3 fish oils only; over-the-counter preparations are also available, but are not FDA-approved formulations. mCan only be prescribed through the FDA's Risk Evaluation and Mitigation Strategy (REMS). *Best taken with meals.

cholestyramine, which are resins that need to be mixed into water. A potential added advantage of bile acid sequestrants is a lowering of A1C levels by ~0.5%, although colesevelam is the only agent that is currently approved by the U.S. Food and Drug Administration (FDA) for glucose lowering.[33] The new class of subcutaneously injected proprotein convertase subtilisin/kexin type-9 (PCSK9) inhibitors not only lower LDL cholesterol to a degree similar to high-intensity statins and appear to be well tolerated, but have also been added to background statin therapy, potentially achieving unprecedented degrees of cumulative LDL cholesterol lowering.[34] However, their cost is currently prohibitive and at present should be reserved for high-risk patients with proven intolerance to multiple statins, or who require substantial LDL cholesterol reductions that are not otherwise achievable. Other medication choices that principally lower TG levels (fibrates, nicotinic acid, high-dose omega-3 fish oils) may also help to lower LDL cholesterol, but will be discussed later in this chapter.

HYPERTRIGLYCERIDEMIA AND ASCVD

In diabetes, elevated TG levels are commonly seen. They are clearly associated with increased ASCVD risk,[35,36] but much of that association can be attributed to other ASCVD risk factors that are tightly correlated with high TG levels. These risk factors include higher levels of apolipoprotein B–containing particles (i.e., mostly VLDL particles that also carry cholesterol as well as TGs), lower levels of HDL cholesterol, LDL particles that are smaller and more proatherogenic (independent of the actual LDL cholesterol level), and the central obesity and insulin resistance that characterizes most patients with type 2 diabetes,[36] all of which also contribute to higher ASCVD risk. Thus, high TG levels are clearly a marker of a high ASCVD risk profile, but whether they also directly confer some lesser but still independent contribution to ASCVD risk remains less clear.

Fibrates, nicotinic acid, and high-dose omega-3 fish oils are available as strong TG-lowering agents (Table 4.4); high-intensity statin treatment can also lower TG levels to some extent, although their principal action is to lower LDL cholesterol. Clinical trial evidence exists to support ASCVD event reduction with fibrates and niacin, albeit not as extensive as that of statins, and much of it from before the modern era of statins; no good evidence yet exists for high-dose fish oils. The Helsinki Heart Study showed that gemfibrozil significantly reduced ASCVD events in high-risk men,[37] although LDL cholesterol was also significantly reduced. A subsequent analysis of this study found that in the overweight subgroup with TG ≥203 mg/dL and HDL cholesterol <42 mg/dL at baseline (i.e., the typical profile of patients with diabetes), the ASCVD event reductions were even more pronounced.[38] The Veterans Affairs High-Density Lipoprotein Intervention Trial (VA-HIT) found that gemfibrozil significantly lowered ASCVD events in high-risk men without significantly reducing LDL cholesterol[39] and that the relative risk reduction was even greater in the subgroups of patients with high fasting insulin levels (indicating insulin resistance) and with established diabetes.[40] The large Fenofibrate Intervention and Event Lowering in Diabetes (FIELD) study showed a significant reduction in nonfatal MIs with fenofibrate but nonsignificant changes in coronary or total mortality (although curiously, progression of diabetic retinopathy and albuminuria were also reduced).[41] However, a subgroup analysis of those patients with marked hypertriglyceridemia (TGs ≥204 mg/dL and HDL cholesterol <40 mg/dL for men and <50 mg/dL for women) had the greatest benefit in ASCVD risk reduction.[42] As for nicotinic acid, in the niacin arm of the Coronary Drug Project, the risk of recurrent MIs and strokes in high-risk men was significantly reduced after 6.2 years, and total mortality was reduced after a total of 15 years of follow-up.[43] Thus, there is interventional trial evidence that fibrates and niacin reduce ASCVD events and particularly for fibrates in insulin-resistant (or diabetic) patients manifesting high TG and low HDL cholesterol levels.

In the modern era of widespread statin use, studies have also examined the utility of adding fibrates or nicotinic acid to background statin use. The lipid-lowering arm of the Action to Control Cardiovascular Risk in Diabetes study (ACCORD-LIPID)[44] was not able to demonstrate further reduction of any ASCVD outcome measure when fenofibrate was added to simvastatin, despite favorable changes in TG and HDL cholesterol levels. However, a trend towards reducing major ASCVD events was noted in the subgroup of patients with TGs ≥204 mg/dL and HDL cholesterol ≤34 mg/dL.[44] The Atherothrombosis Intervention in Metabolic Syndrome with Low HDL/High Triglycerides: Impact on Global Health Outcomes (AIM-HIGH) study that enrolled patients with established ASCVD and baseline TGs ≥150 mg/dL and HDL cholesterol <40 mg/dL for men and <50 mg/dL for women (approximately 33% with diabetes), failed to demonstrate further reduction of any ASCVD outcome measure when extended-release niacin was added to background statin therapy.[45] However, a subsequent analysis of patients at the extreme tertiles for TG (≥198 mg/dL) and HDL cholesterol (<33 mg/dL) found a trend towards a reduction in ASCVD outcomes.[46] Also, the large Heart Protection Study 2–Treatment of HDL to Reduce the Incidence of Vascular Events (HPS2-THRIVE) study of extended-release niacin (formulated together with a flushing inhibitor), when added to background statin therapy in patients with prior ASCVD (approximately 32% with diabetes), not only failed to show a significant benefit on major ASCVD outcome measures, but also noted an excess of serious adverse events.[47] Specifically, there was a 32% higher rate of new-onset diabetes, a 55% increase in disturbances of glucose control that were regarded as serious (most of which required hospitalization), as well as higher rates of gastrointestinal and musculoskeletal side effects (including a fourfold higher rate of myopathy), and an unexpected increase in infections and bleeding events.[47] And unlike prior studies, a subgroup analysis of those patients with TG >151 mg/dL and HDL cholesterol <40 mg/dL in men or <51 mg/dL in women failed to show any trend towards a significant ASCVD reduction. Therefore, while adding fibrates or nicotinic acid to a statin can produce favorable lipid changes, the evidence that the ASCVD benefits outweigh the risks is currently insufficient (and potentially *unfavorable* in the case of extended-release niacin). Although there might still be some unproven benefit for those patients with particularly high TG and low HDL cholesterol levels, any decision to add these agents should be made based on individualized judgment of the risks and benefits. To date, there are no studies of sufficient quality that examine the addition of high-dose omega-3 fish oils to statins to reduce ASCVD outcomes.

HYPERTRIGLYCERIDEMIA AND PANCREATITIS

Notwithstanding the foregoing considerations of ASCVD risk, when TG levels rise to extreme levels (e.g., ≥1,000 mg/dL), the more immediate risk of precipitating an attack of acute pancreatitis takes priority over any longer-term risk of increasing ASCVD events. TG elevations to this extent occur uncommonly, but except for patients with a known primary (inherited) defect in lipolysis, most cases are usually seen in the setting of severe obesity, uncontrolled diabetes, alcohol abuse, or medications that exacerbate TG levels (e.g., glucocorticoids, estrogens) in individuals who are uniquely susceptible to such factors.[48] Extreme hypertriglyceridemia to this extent reflects chylomicron retention resulting from a saturated lipolytic system, leading to an acceleration of TG elevations that can go far higher than just 1,000 mg/dL. Patients may be asymptomatic (if acute pancreatitis has not occurred), but may manifest cutaneous eruptive xanthomata or lipemia retinalis on fundoscopy; blood may also be visibly lipemic during phlebotomy. The TG threshold at which acute pancreatitis occurs is highly variable, but in those with prior attacks of pancreatitis, a recurrent attack can occur with TG levels even between 500 and 1,000 mg/dL. No rigorous clinical trials have tested the efficacy of the recommended treatment approach outlined below or any specific TG-lowering medications, or that have compared different treatment strategies for treating or preventing hypertriglyceridemia-associated pancreatitis. However, anecdotal clinical experience indicates that the recommended treatment approach outlined below for extreme hypertriglyceridemia is effective.

PRINCIPLES OF HYPERTRIGLYCERIDEMIA TREATMENT

If the TG level is extremely high (e.g., ≥1,000 mg/dL, or ≥500 mg/dL in the setting of suspected pancreatitis), the TG level should be lowered urgently to reduce pancreatitis risk. If there is also clinical suspicion of acute pancreatitis already occurring, the patient should be managed as a medical emergency and hospitalized. In the subsequent transition back toward outpatient management, or for initial aggressive outpatient management in asymptomatic individuals without acute pancreatitis, careful attention must be paid to all factors that can exacerbate TG levels. These steps include strict dietary restriction of fats and simple carbohydrates (including fructose-containing or sugar-sweetened beverages), avoiding alcohol and any medications that can elevate TG levels, and optimizing glucose control. Effective adjunctive TG-lowering medications (i.e., fibrates, nicotinic acid, or high-dose omega-3 fish oils, but *not statins*, which have a more limited effect on lowering TG levels) should be started as a first-line monotherapy choice, and strict medication adherence should be emphasized. There are no specific TG targets recommended for the effective treatment or prevention of acute pancreatitis; treatment should generally aim to keep the TG levels as low as possible.

Once TG levels no longer put the patient at risk of pancreatitis (e.g., 200–500 mg/dL), it should be remembered that the longer-term risk of increased ASCVD events still remains a concern when TG levels are only moderately elevated. In such patients, there is still a role for statins. In this situation, it would be ideal if co-management of all other contributions to the extreme hypertriglyceridemia (e.g., better diabetes control, dietary optimization, discontinuation of alcohol and any offending medications) can eventually reduce the TG level sufficiently to permit reduction or discontinuation of the TG-lowering agent, such that a statin can be substituted instead of having to be added. However, if the TG-lowering agent cannot be discontinued, and the patient's risk profile still requires that a statin be added, it should be added cautiously (as discussed below). At our institution, we choose fenofibrate for asymptomatic patients with TG levels ≥1,000 mg/dL to reduce pancreatitis risk; TG levels are then followed monthly while concurrent factors are addressed in an attempt to eventually discontinue the fenofibrate, if possible, while keeping TG levels <1,000 mg/dL.

ATP-III originally recognized the ASCVD risk conferred by the moderately high-TG, low-HDL cholesterol dyslipidemia phenotype (that is independent of LDL cholesterol levels) and recommended that this risk should be managed as a secondary target of ASCVD risk reduction, after the primary target, LDL cholesterol, has been optimized.[18] Non–HDL cholesterol was recommended as a surrogate marker of this combined lipid phenotype:

Non–HDL cholesterol = Total cholesterol – HDL cholesterol

This measure encompasses the cholesterol content of all pro-atherogenic lipid particles, which for most individuals consists predominantly of VLDL cholesterol and LDL cholesterol. Because LDL cholesterol should have been optimized as the first priority of lipid control, the non–HDL cholesterol level therefore closely reflects the remaining VLDL cholesterol (i.e., the potential atherogenicity of the TG-containing VLDL particles remaining in fasting plasma). The relative stability of the non–HDL cholesterol measure compared to the TG level (since TG levels can be highly labile even on fasting samples), its reliability even in the non-fasting state (since it does not depend on having to measure a fasting TG level, and since cholesterol measures are much less affected by non-fasting), and the fact that it can be calculated on every lipid panel and therefore entails no additional costs, all make non–HDL cholesterol a more ideal target of therapy than TG or HDL cholesterol levels. There is also evidence that non–HDL cholesterol may be a better predictor of ASCVD risk and a more effective target of therapy than LDL cholesterol.[49]

ATP-III recommends that after LDL cholesterol has been treated to goal (i.e., <100 mg/dL for all diabetes patients, or <70 mg/dL for diabetes patients with overt ASCVD), for those patients with fasting TGs ≥200 mg/dL, the non–HDL cholesterol should be calculated, and if it is not controlled below its respective target, then treatment should be further intensified until both the LDL cholesterol and non–HDL cholesterol targets have been achieved.[18] Non–HDL cholesterol targets are always 30 mg/dL above the corresponding LDL cholesterol target for a given patient's risk profile; hence, for diabetes patients with LDL cholesterol targets <100 mg/dL or <70 mg/dL, the respective non–HDL cholesterol targets should be <130 mg/dL or <100 mg/dL. It should be noted that the ACC/AHA guidelines do not advocate the use of non–HDL cholesterol levels at all in making treatment decisions. At our institution, after applying the fixed-dose statin strategy discussed above, we additionally pursue both LDL cholesterol and non–HDL cholesterol targets of ATP-III for maximal ASCVD risk reduction.

In addition to dietary and lifestyle measures that help to control TG levels as discussed above, TG-related ASCVD risk reduction should additionally focus on overall caloric balance and weight control (i.e., control of total dietary fat, simple carbohydrates, and total calories, as well as increasing regular physical activity), since obesity is associated with both hypertriglyceridemia and ASCVD risk (and often elevated non–HDL cholesterol as well). In terms of drug therapy, statins are still the preferred choice for control of non–HDL cholesterol (since LDL cholesterol is a component of the non–HDL cholesterol level, further lowering of LDL cholesterol will correspondingly lower non–HDL cholesterol). Thus, progressive intensification of statins is still the most evidence-based initial strategy to achieve non–HDL cholesterol goals. And just as with the pursuit of LDL cholesterol goals, once a maximum dose (or maximum-tolerated dose) of a single statin is reached, under our approach used at our institution, a suitable non-statin agent should be added; ezetimibe, bile acid sequestrants, and PCSK9 inhibitors may all be considered.

If these options fail or are not tolerated, TG-lowering agents such as fibrates or nicotinic acid (Table 4.4) may also be alternative considerations to lower non–HDL cholesterol (since lowering TG-containing VLDL particles will also lower non–HDL cholesterol), bearing in mind the lack of good ASCVD outcomes evidence supporting such drug combinations. At our institution, we would consider adding such agents, going beyond the ADA recommendations. There are also cautions that should be observed when adding fibrates or nicotinic acid to statins. Fibrates effectively lower TG and raise HDL cholesterol levels and, in most cases, also modestly lower LDL cholesterol levels. When used by themselves, the same cautions that apply to statins should be observed (e.g., ALT elevations, myositis), along with an increased risk of cholelithiasis and severe renal insufficiency as a contraindication. However, when used in combination with statins, the risks of statin toxicity are magnified[29]; in such cases, a wise precaution would be to start regular monitoring for ALT elevations and myositis (e.g., every 1–2 months for the first year of combination therapy). In addition, fenofibrate and not gemfibrozil should be used, since the risk of rhabdomyolysis is some 15-fold higher when gemfibrozil is added compared to fenofibrate.[50] However, evidence does support fenofibrate further lowering ASCVD risk when added to a statin in patients with TG levels ≥204 mg/dL and HDL cholesterol levels ≤34 mg/dL.[26] Fenofibrate can also increase ezetimibe levels, so that combination should ideally be avoided.

Niacin preparations commonly cause dose-dependent flushing, pruritus, and GI upset after each dose (which may be less with the extended-release preparations) and require gradual up-titration of the dose, but these symptoms often subside with ongoing use. Aspirin (325 mg) taken 30 min before each dose, as well as avoidance of alcohol and spicy foods, can lessen the severity of the flushing. Niacin can also cause ALT elevations and hyperuricemia and, at higher doses, may worsen glucose control. As monotherapy, niacin may reduce ASCVD risk in high-risk individuals.[43] However, when added to statins, the risk of hepatotoxicity increases as it does with fibrates, so regular monitoring for ALT elevations would also be a wise precaution.[51] In addition, there is no evidence of further ASCVD risk reduction that justifies the increased risk of adverse events when niacin is added to a statin.[45,47]

At our institution, to further pursue the non–HDL cholesterol target, we opt for the addition of fenofibrate when the addition of ezetimibe has failed to achieve targets because of the poor tolerance of bile acid sequestrants and the current unavailability of PCSK9 inhibitors. However, we may not necessarily add it until non–HDL cholesterol is ≥160 mg/dL, based on the potential fibrate-statin interaction and based on data from a pooled analysis of four large population cohorts that found that the risk of ASCVD events in both diabetic and nondiabetic patients were not any higher at a level of 130–159 mg/dL compared to <130 mg/dL; that is, the risk did not increase until the non–HDL cholesterol level was ≥160 mg/dL.[52] Although this analysis was not based on interventional trial data, no clinical trial data exist to support the superiority of one non–HDL cholesterol target over another. Also, instead of gradually titrating the fenofibrate dose upwards, we simply prescribe the maximum dose of the available fenofibrate formulation (listed in Table 4.4). Once the patient's LDL cholesterol and non–HDL cholesterol goals have both been achieved, follow-up lipid panels are obtained every 3–4 months thereafter to monitor for ongoing medication adherence and maintenance of targets, with further intensification of treatment as needed.

The omega-3 polyunsaturated fatty acids eicosapentaenoic acid (EPA) and docosahexaenoic acid (DHA) (i.e., the marine fish oils), when taken in doses of 3–4 g daily, can substantially lower TG levels. However, LDL cholesterol levels may also increase modestly (attributable to the DHA component, which can be mitigated by concurrent statin use), so the effects of such doses on ASCVD risk remain unclear. There are no clinical trials of sufficient quality examining the ASCVD effects of such TG-lowering doses. Many earlier studies using lower, supplemental doses of omega-3 fish oils (e.g., up to 1–2 g of EPA + DHA daily) have suggested a modest ASCVD event reduction overall,[53] but the recent omega-3 fatty acids arm of the Outcome Reduction with an Initial Glargine Intervention (ORIGIN) trial in diabetic and prediabetic patients, 54% of whom were taking background statins at baseline, found no significant ASCVD protection whatsoever.[54] This evidence, together with other recent trials, suggests that any ASCVD benefit with fish oils may be insignificant when compared to that of statins, which are now widely used.[55,56] Omega-3 fish oils are generally well tolerated, even at high doses. Over-the-counter preparations, while less expensive, are not FDA-regulated, so their purity and consistency of EPA and DHA content cannot be guaranteed. In contrast, pharmacological omega-3 preparations (Table 4.4) are more concentrated (thus requiring fewer capsules to achieve the high doses) and are FDA-approved as an adjunct to diet for the treatment of TG levels ≥500 mg/dL. Thus, while high-dose omega-3 fish oils may have a role in treating severe hypertriglyceridemia and pancreatitis risk, their role for ASCVD prevention, either as monotherapy or added to statins, remains to be established.

DYSLIPIDEMIA ALGORITHM

This algorithm is used at our institution, and recommends treatments beyond those of the ADA recommendations. It is also not intended to be a comprehensive guide to the management of lipid disorders. Referral to appropriate lipid specialists should be considered for suspected genetic dyslipidemias or other severe or complex lipid disorders.

1. Measure fasting baseline lipid panel.
2. All diabetes patients ≥40 years old should be taking a statin regardless of baseline LDL cholesterol concentration; appropriate dietary and lifestyle measures should be reinforced at every visit.
3. Goal level of LDL cholesterol is <100 mg/dL, or <70 mg/dL if patient has overt ASCVD.
4. Initial doses of atorvastatin or rosuvastatin (if patient not already taking a statin) are shown in Table 4.3.
5. Measure lipid panel 1 month after starting or changing a statin dose. If LDL cholesterol level is not at goal, double the statin dose and reassess LDL cholesterol level 1 month later; continue to double the statin dose every month until LDL cholesterol goal level is achieved, a maximum allowable dose is reached, or statin intolerance occurs. If a maximum allowable dose is reached or statin intolerance occurs and LDL cholesterol level is still not at goal, add ezetimibe, a bile acid sequestrant, or a PCSK9 inhibitor agent to achieve LDL cholesterol goal.
6. If patient is already on another statin and the LDL cholesterol level is already at goal, maintain this statin at its present dose.
7. If patient is already on another statin and the LDL cholesterol level is not at goal, convert to the appropriate atorvastatin or rosuvastatin dose for the patient's risk profile (Table 4.3). Measure lipid panel 1 month later. If LDL cholesterol level is not at goal, double the statin dose and reassess LDL cholesterol level 1 month later; continue to double statin dose until LDL cholesterol goal level is achieved, a maximum allowable dose is reached, or statin intolerance occurs. If a maximum allowable dose is reached or statin intolerance occurs and LDL cholesterol level is still not at goal, add ezetimibe, a bile acid sequestrant, or a PCSK9 inhibitor to achieve LDL cholesterol goal.
8. If initial TG concentration is ≥1,000 mg/dL, also start fenofibrate at its maximum allowable dose, and emphasize appropriate dietary and lifestyle restrictions; re-measure TG concentration in 1 month:
   a) If TG concentration remains ≥1,000 mg/dL, continue fenofibrate, re-emphasize appropriate dietary and lifestyle restrictions, and consider the use of nicotinic acid or high-dose omega-3 fish oils.
   b) If TG concentration <1,000 mg/dL, discontinue fenofibrate and re-measure TG concentration in 1 month; if TG concentration increases back to ≥1,000 mg/dL, restart fenofibrate at maximum allowable dose as before and measure TG concentration in 1 month; if it still remains ≥1,000 mg/dL, consider the use of nicotinic acid or high-dose omega-3 fish oils.

9. Once LDL cholesterol is at goal, if TG concentration is 200–999 mg/dL, calculate non–HDL cholesterol; if this value is >130 mg/dL (or >100 mg/dL in patients with overt ASCVD), continue to double statin dose every month until the appropriate non–HDL cholesterol goal is reached, a maximum allowable dose is reached, or statin intolerance occurs. If a maximum allowable dose is reached or statin intolerance occurs and non–HDL cholesterol level is still not at goal, add ezetimibe.

10. If the patient reaches maximum allowable or maximum tolerable statin doses plus ezetimibe, there are two possibilities to consider. If the TG concentration is >200 mg/dL *and* the HDL cholesterol concentration is <35 mg/dL, consider either fenofibrate or a PCSK9 inhibitor. If *either* or *both* the TG and HDL concentrations do not meet these criteria, consider a PCSK9 inhibitor. For the reasons discussed in the text, a non–HDL cholesterol threshold of ≥160 mg/dL is used before adding a maximal allowable dose of fenofibrate (because of the potential interactions with statins and ezetimibe) or a PCSK9 inhibitor (because of injections being required and/or the cost).

11. Once LDL cholesterol and non–HDL cholesterol, if TG concentrations are 200–999 mg/dL, are both at goal, measure lipids every 3–4 months to assess compliance. Intensify treatment as described above if lipids increase above goal levels (and patients are taking their lipid medications).

REFERENCES

1. Haffner SM, Lehto S, Ronnemaa T, Pyorala K, Laakso M. Mortality from coronary heart disease in subjects with type 2 diabetes and in nondiabetic subjects with and without prior myocardial infarction. *N Engl J Med* 1998;339:229–234

2. Malmberg K, Yusuf S, Gerstein HC, et al. Impact of diabetes on long-term prognosis in patients with unstable angina and non-Q-wave myocardial infarction: results of the OASIS (Organization to Assess Strategies for Ischemic Syndromes) Registry. *Circulation* 2000;102:1014–1019

3. Mukamal KJ, Nesto RW, Cohen MC, et al. Impact of diabetes on long-term survival after acute myocardial infarction: comparability of risk with prior myocardial infarction. *Diabetes Care* 2001;24:1422–1427

4. Baigent C, Keech A, Kearney PM, et al. Efficacy and safety of cholesterol-lowering treatment: prospective meta-analysis of data from 90,056 participants in 14 randomised trials of statins. *Lancet* 2005;366:1267–1278

5. Baigent C, Blackwell L, Emberson J, et al. Efficacy and safety of more intensive lowering of LDL cholesterol: a meta-analysis of data from 170,000 participants in 26 randomised trials. *Lancet* 2010;376:1670–1681

6. Mihaylova B, Emberson J, Blackwell L, et al. The effects of lowering LDL cholesterol with statin therapy in people at low risk of vascular disease: meta-analysis of individual data from 27 randomised trials. *Lancet* 2012;380:581–590

7. Colhoun HM, Betteridge DJ, Durrington PN, et al. Primary prevention of cardiovascular disease with atorvastatin in type 2 diabetes in the Collaborative Atorvastatin Diabetes Study (CARDS): multicentre randomised placebo-controlled trial. *Lancet* 2004;364:685–696

8. Pyorala K, Pedersen TR, Kjekshus J, et al. Cholesterol lowering with simvastatin improves prognosis of diabetic patients with coronary heart disease. A subgroup analysis of the Scandinavian Simvastatin Survival Study (4S). *Diabetes Care* 1997;20:614–620

9. Goldberg RB, Mellies MJ, Sacks FM, et al; the Care Investigators. Cardiovascular events and their reduction with pravastatin in diabetic and glucose-intolerant myocardial infarction survivors with average cholesterol levels: subgroup analyses in the cholesterol and recurrent events (CARE) trial. *Circulation* 1998;98:2513–2519

10. Serruys PW, de Feyter P, Macaya C, et al. Fluvastatin for prevention of cardiac events following successful first percutaneous coronary intervention: a randomized controlled trial. *JAMA* 2002;287:3215–3222

11. Athyros VG, Papageorgiou AA, Mercouris BR, et al. Treatment with atorvastatin to the National Cholesterol Educational Program goal versus 'usual' care in secondary coronary heart disease prevention: the GREek Atorvastatin and Coronary-heart-disease Evaluation (GREACE) study. *Curr Med Res Opin* 2002;18:220–228

12. Collins R, Armitage J, Parish S, et al. MRC/BHF Heart Protection Study of cholesterol-lowering with simvastatin in 5963 people with diabetes: a randomised placebo-controlled trial. *Lancet* 2003;361:2005–2016

13. Sever PS, Poulter NR, Dahlof B, et al. Reduction in cardiovascular events with atorvastatin in 2,532 patients with type 2 diabetes: Anglo-Scandinavian Cardiac Outcomes Trial—Lipid-Lowering Arm (ASCOT-LLA). *Diabetes Care* 2005;28:1151–1157

14. Shepherd J, Barter P, Carmena R, et al. Effect of lowering LDL cholesterol substantially below currently recommended levels in patients with coronary heart disease and diabetes: the Treating to New Targets (TNT) study. *Diabetes Care* 2006;29:1220–1226

15. Tajima N, Kurata H, Nakaya N, et al. Pravastatin reduces the risk for cardiovascular disease in Japanese hypercholesterolemic patients with impaired fasting glucose or diabetes: diabetes subanalysis of the Management of Elevated Cholesterol in the Primary Prevention Group of Adult Japanese (MEGA) Study. *Atherosclerosis* 2008;199:455–462

16. Callahan A, Amarenco P, Goldstein LB, et al. Risk of stroke and cardiovascular events after ischemic stroke or transient ischemic attack in patients with type 2 diabetes or metabolic syndrome: secondary analysis of the Stroke Prevention by Aggressive Reduction in Cholesterol Levels (SPARCL) trial. *Arch Neurol* 2011;68:1245–1251

17. Kearney PM, Blackwell L, Collins R, et al. Efficacy of cholesterol-lowering therapy in 18,686 people with diabetes in 14 randomised trials of statins: a meta-analysis. *Lancet* 2008;371:117–125

18. Expert Panel on Detection, Evaluation, and Treatment of High Blood Cholesterol In Adults. Executive summary of the third report of the National Cholesterol Education Program (NCEP) Expert Panel on Detection, Evaluation, and Treatment of High Blood Cholesterol in Adults (Adult Treatment Panel III). *JAMA* 2001;285:2486–2497

19. Grundy SM, Cleeman JI, Merz CN, et al. Implications of recent clinical trials for the National Cholesterol Education Program Adult Treatment Panel III guidelines. *Circulation* 2004;110:227–239

20. Stone NJ, Robinson JG, Lichtenstein AH, et al. 2013 ACC/AHA guideline on the treatment of blood cholesterol to reduce atherosclerotic cardiovascular risk in adults: a report of the American College of Cardiology/American Heart Association Task Force on Practice Guidelines. *Circulation* 2014;129(25 Suppl. 2):S1–S45

21. Law MR, Wald NJ, Thompson SG. By how much and how quickly does reduction in serum cholesterol concentration lower risk of ischaemic heart disease? *BMJ* 1994;308:367–372

22. Law MR, Wald NJ. An ecological study of serum cholesterol and ischaemic heart disease between 1950 and 1990. *Eur J Clin Nutr* 1994;48:305–325

23. Law MR, Wald NJ, Rudnicka AR. Quantifying effect of statins on low density lipoprotein cholesterol, ischaemic heart disease, and stroke: systematic review and meta-analysis. *BMJ* 2003;326:1423

24. Egan BM, Li J, Qanungo S, Wolfman TE. Blood pressure and cholesterol control in hypertensive hypercholesterolemic patients: National Health and Nutrition Examination Surveys 1988–2010. *Circulation* 2013;128:29–41

25. Roth GA, Fihn SD, Mokdad AH, et al. High total serum cholesterol, medication coverage and therapeutic control: an analysis of national health examination survey data from eight countries. *Bull World Health Org* 2011;89:92–101

26. American Diabetes Association. Cardiovascular disease and risk management. *Diabetes Care* 2016;39(Suppl. 1):S60–S71

27. Mora S, Rifai N, Buring JE, Ridker PM. Comparison of LDL cholesterol concentrations by Friedewald calculation and direct measurement in relation to cardiovascular events in 27,331 women. *Clin Chem* 2009;55:888–894

28. Mangravite LM, Thorn CF, Krauss RM. Clinical implications of pharmacogenomics of statin treatment. *Pharmacogenomics J* 2006;6:360–374

29. Golomb BA, Evans MA. Statin adverse effects: a review of the literature and evidence for a mitochondrial mechanism. *Am J Cardiovasc Drugs* 2008;8:373–418

30. Cannon CP, Blazing MA, Giugliano RP, et al. Ezetimibe added to statin therapy after acute coronary syndromes. *N Engl J Med* 2015;372:2387–2397

31. LaRosa J. Review of clinical studies of bile acid sequestrants for lowering plasma lipid levels. *Cardiology* 1989;76(Suppl. 1):55–61

32. Lipid Research Clinics Program. The Lipid Research Clinics Coronary Primary Prevention Trial results. I. Reduction in incidence of coronary heart disease. *JAMA* 1984;251:351–364

33. Hansen M, Sonne DP, Knop FK. Bile acid sequestrants: glucose-lowering mechanisms and efficacy in type 2 diabetes. *Curr Diab Rep* 2014;14:482

34. Dadu RT, Ballantyne CM. Lipid lowering with PCSK9 inhibitors. *Nat Rev Cardiol* 2014;11:563–575

35. Sarwar N, Danesh J, Eiriksdottir G, et al. Triglycerides and the risk of coronary heart disease: 10,158 incident cases among 262,525 participants in 29 western prospective studies. *Circulation* 2007;115:450–458

36. Miller M, Stone NJ, Ballantyne C, et al. Triglycerides and cardiovascular disease: a scientific statement from the American Heart Association. *Circulation* 2011;123:2292–2333

37. Frick MH, Elo O, Haapa K, et al. Helsinki Heart Study: primary-prevention trial with gemfibrozil in middle-aged men with dyslipidemia: safety of treatment, changes in risk factors, and incidence of coronary heart disease. *N Engl J Med* 1987;317:1237–1245

38. Tenkanen L, Manttari M, Manninen V. Some coronary risk factors related to the insulin resistance syndrome and treatment with gemfibrozil: experience from the Helsinki Heart Study. *Circulation* 1995;92:1779–1785

39. Rubins HB, Robins SJ, Collins D, et al.; Veterans Affairs High-Density Lipoprotein Cholesterol Intervention Trial Study Group. Gemfibrozil for the secondary prevention of coronary heart disease in men with low levels of high-density lipoprotein cholesterol. *N Engl J Med* 1999;341:410–418

40. Rubins HB, Robins SJ, Collins D, et al. Diabetes, plasma insulin, and cardiovascular disease: subgroup analysis from the Department of Veterans Affairs High-Density Lipoprotein Intervention Trial (VA-HIT). *Arch Intern Med* 2002;162:2597–2604

41. Keech A, Simes RJ, Barter P, et al. Effects of long-term fenofibrate therapy on cardiovascular events in 9795 people with type 2 diabetes mellitus (the FIELD study): randomised controlled trial. *Lancet* 2005;366:1849–1861

42. Scott R, O'Brien R, Fulcher G, et al. Effects of fenofibrate treatment on cardiovascular disease risk in 9,795 individuals with type 2 diabetes and various components of the metabolic syndrome: the Fenofibrate Intervention and Event Lowering in Diabetes (FIELD) study. *Diabetes Care* 2009;32:493–498

43. Canner PL, Berge KG, Wenger NK, et al. Fifteen year mortality in Coronary Drug Project patients: long-term benefit with niacin. *J Am Coll Cardiol* 1986;8:1245–1255

44. Ginsberg HN, Elam MB, Lovato LC, et al. Effects of combination lipid therapy in type 2 diabetes mellitus. *N Engl J Med* 2010;362:1563–1574

45. Boden WE, Probstfield JL, Anderson T, et al. Niacin in patients with low HDL cholesterol levels receiving intensive statin therapy. *N Engl J Med* 2011;365:2255–2267

46. Guyton JR, Slee AE, Anderson T, et al. Relationship of lipoproteins to cardiovascular events: the AIM-HIGH Trial (Atherothrombosis Intervention in Metabolic Syndrome With Low HDL/High Triglycerides and Impact on Global Health Outcomes). *J Am Coll Cardiol* 2013;62:1580–1584

47. Landray MJ, Haynes R, Hopewell JC, et al. Effects of extended-release niacin with laropiprant in high-risk patients. *N Engl J Med* 2014;371:203–212

48. Brahm AJ, Hegele RA. Chylomicronaemia: current diagnosis and future therapies. *Nat Rev Endocrinol* 2015;11:352–362

49. Ramjee V, Sperling LS, Jacobson TA. Non-high-density lipoprotein cholesterol versus apolipoprotein B in cardiovascular risk stratification: do the math. *J Am Coll Cardiol* 2011;58:457–463

50. Jones PH, Davidson MH. Reporting rate of rhabdomyolysis with fenofibrate + statin versus gemfibrozil + any statin. *Am J Cardiol* 2005;95:120–122

51. Creider JC, Hegele RA, Joy TR. Niacin: another look at an underutilized lipid-lowering medication. *Nat Rev Endocrinol* 2012;8:517–528

52. Liu J, Sempos C, Donahue RP, et al. Joint distribution of non-HDL and LDL cholesterol and coronary heart disease risk prediction among individuals with and without diabetes. *Diabetes Care* 2005;28:1916–1921

53. Artham SM, Lavie CJ, Milani RV, et al. Fish oil in primary and secondary cardiovascular prevention. *Ochsner J* 2008;8:49–60

54. Bosch J, Gerstein HC, Dagenais GR, et al. n-3 fatty acids and cardiovascular outcomes in patients with dysglycemia. *N Engl J Med* 2012;367:309–318

55. Kromhout D, Yasuda S, Geleijnse JM, Shimokawa H. Fish oil and omega-3 fatty acids in cardiovascular disease: do they really work? *Eur Heart J* 2012;33:436–443

56. Eussen SR, Geleijnse JM, Giltay EJ, et al. Effects of n-3 fatty acids on major cardiovascular events in statin users and non-users with a history of myocardial infarction. *Eur Heart J* 2012;33:1582–1588

Chapter 5
Hypertension

There is a direct and continuous relationship between higher blood pressure (BP) and higher atherosclerotic cardiovascular disease (ASCVD) risk, down to BP levels as low as 115/75 mmHg.[1] As discussed in Chapter 1, numerous comparative trials have demonstrated the benefits of BP control on macrovascular complications in individuals with diabetes, with more intensive BP lowering resulting in greater lowering of ASCVD and/or stroke events.[2-8] However, there may not be any further ASCVD benefit in lowering BP below 140/90 mmHg.[7-10] In the Systolic Hypertension in the Elderly Program (SHEP) study, although the relative reduction of ASCVD events is similar between diabetic and nondiabetic patients, the baseline ASCVD risk in individuals with diabetes is higher than that of nondiabetic individuals, so in terms of absolute numbers of ASCVD events prevented, the reduction is greater in individuals with diabetes.[2] In addition, in the Systolic Hypertension in Europe (Syst-Eur) study, while the diabetes subjects had the same magnitude of BP reduction as the nondiabetic subjects, there was a substantially greater percent reduction of ASCVD and stroke events, ASCVD mortality, and overall mortality in the subjects with diabetes compared to the nondiabetic subjects.[5]

As discussed in Chapter 1, BP lowering also has beneficial effects on the microvascular complications of diabetic retinopathy and nephropathy. Long-term BP reduction in diabetes slows the progressive decline in glomerular filtration rate (GFR) and the progressive rise in albuminuria,[6,11,12] particularly at earlier stages when albuminuria is lower.[6] In the Action to Control Cardiovascular Risk in Diabetes (ACCORD)-BP Study, more intensive BP control reduced albuminuria more effectively than less intensive control.[8] In the UK Prospective Diabetes Study (UKPDS), the proportion of individuals with albuminuria (defined as ≥50 mg/L) was slightly lower with intensive compared to less intensive BP control after 6 years of treatment, although the differences in that study were not significant with respect to shorter or longer timeframes, albuminuria ≥300 mg/L, the incidence of renal failure, or deaths due to renal failure.[3] In general, there is stronger interventional trial evidence supporting benefits of more aggressive BP control on albuminuria as a marker of diabetic nephropathy than on declining renal function or progression to end-stage renal failure. With respect to diabetic retinopathy, one population-based cohort study found that over 9 years of follow-up, risk of incident diabetic retinopathy increased by 30% with every 10-mmHg increase in baseline systolic BP, but that treatment with anti-hypertension agents reduced that incidence by 50%.[13] The UKPDS, which achieved a mean intensive BP of 144/82 mmHg versus a less intensive level of 154/87 mmHg, found that intensive BP control from a median of 4.5 years onwards slowed the worsening retinopathy scores by 25–34% and, over a median of 7.5 years, slowed vision deterioration by 47% compared to less intensive BP control.[3] However, in the ACCORD Eye Study, even more intensive BP control targeting systolic BP to <120 mmHg versus <140 mmHg failed to reduce the progression of diabetic retinopathy any further.[14]

PRINCIPLES OF HYPERTENSION TREATMENT

Blood pressure should be measured at every routine visit for patients with diabetes. As is recommended for the general population, an appropriately trained individual should perform BP measurements in a standardized manner.[15] Specifically, a cuff of appropriate size for the length and circumference of the upper arm should be used on a seated patient with the arm supported at the level of the heart and after at least 5 minutes of seated rest. Elevated BP readings should be repeated at least once on another day to verify the persistence of the elevation before beginning treatment.

The American Diabetes Association (ADA) recommends that BP in patients with diabetes should be controlled to below 140/90 mmHg, based on evidence of reductions in ASCVD, stroke, and renal outcomes[16]; lifestyle modifications are indicated for any BP >120/80 mmHg, and pharmacological agents are recommended for any confirmed office BP reading >140/90 mmHg.[16] More intensive control to lower BP targets only produces a small additional reduction in absolute stroke events, no additional reduction in ASCVD outcomes, and an increased risk of adverse events.[9,10] However, the ADA does recommend that if a lower target such as 130/80 mmHg can be achieved without undue treatment burden in patients at higher ASCVD risk, the benefits of doing so may outweigh the risks.[16] This additional recommendation is consistent with the recent Systolic Blood Pressure Intervention Trial (SPRINT) that, while excluding individuals with diabetes, nevertheless showed that more stringent BP control (mean systolic BP of 121 mmHg compared to 136 mmHg) led to a further 25% reduction in composite ASCVD events, including a reduction in all-cause mortality, although rates of serious adverse events were also higher.[17] A more recent meta-analysis of comparative studies, specifically in patients with diabetes, found net benefits for reducing ASCVD and stroke events, end-stage renal disease, and/or all-cause mortality only if the systolic BP before starting treatment was >140 mmHg and the attained BP was 130–140 mmHg. However, there may be net harm for ASCVD mortality if baseline BP was <140 mmHg,[18] suggesting that in patients with diabetes, treatment of systolic B that is already <140 mmHg may not be warranted.

As previously discussed in Chapter 2, reduction of dietary sodium intake has a direct and continuous effect on lowering of BP.[19,20] The ADA currently recommends no more than 2,300 mg sodium per day for all patients with diabetes. A further restriction could be to <1,500 mg daily for hypertensive diabetes patients if such a restriction was realistically achievable,[21] but this more stringent restriction may not be easily followed without affecting overall nutritional quality[22] and may not be associated with further benefits in outcomes.[23,24] Sodium restriction should be part of a prudent overall dietary pattern, such as the Dietary Approaches to Stop Hypertension (DASH) dietary plan,[25] which limits dietary sodium; increases dietary potassium; emphasizes the consumption of fruits, vegetables, and low-fat dairy sources; and limits excessive alcohol intake, all in the context of a balanced intake of total calories and macronutrients from healthy sources.[16] Interventional studies of regular physical activity programs in the general population also show a consistent effect of lowering BP,[26] but such studies in diabetes populations tend to be less consistent; observational studies suggest an association between physical activity and reduced BP, but interventional trials in diabetes populations have produced mixed results.[27] Nevertheless, a regular physical activity program should still be routinely recommended for diabetes patients with hypertension. However, none of these nonpharmacological strategies are liable to produce the same magnitude of BP lowering as pharmacological agents. Thus, the vast majority of patients with hypertension will require one or more anti-hypertension agents to achieve their BP goals.

Traditionally, the stepped-care approach to treat BP to a given target, by starting a single agent and increasing to its maximum dose before adding an additional agent, has been the preferred approach. However, some have instead advocated starting treatment with a combination of two agents at submaximal doses,[28] based on the rationale that dose escalations in the lower part of a drug's dose range are often more effective than dose escalations in the upper part and the fact that most diabetes patients will ultimately require more than one drug to meet their BP goal. However, our hypertension treatment algorithms (which differ slightly from the current ADA recommendations) retain the stepped-care approach for several reasons: *1*) the stepped-care approach simplifies medication regimens as much as possible, since patients with diabetes are usually already taking a multitude of other medications; *2*) they minimize the risk of potential medication side effects and/or interactions by using the minimum number of agents necessary to achieve the BP target; *3*) should unexpected intolerances occur, it would be easier to identify the culprit agent if they had been added one at a time rather than in combinations; *4*) since the algorithm calls for reassessments and dose escalations no less than every month, there is little difference in time saved in achieving the BP goal by starting combinations of agents as compared to adding them sequentially; and *5*) progressive increases of submaximal doses of more than one drug would make for a far more complex treatment algorithm for providers to follow.

There are 11 classes of anti-hypertension drugs currently available in the U.S. Although many head-to-head comparison trials looking at hard outcome measures such as ASCVD, stroke, or mortality events have shown some subtle differences across different medication classes, as a general rule, the benefits are still largely a function of the degree of BP lowering, regardless of the class of agents used.[29] One clear exception has been α_1-adrenergic receptor antagonists; the pivotal Antihypertensive and Lipid-Lowering Treatment to Prevent Heart Attack Trial (ALLHAT) found that the α-blocker doxazosin led to significantly higher rates of ASCVD events compared to all other agents studied (chlorthalidone, lisinopril, amlodipine).[30] But in general, decisions about ideal choices for given situations will usually revolve around other benefits versus risks of each medication class, independent of their effect on BP per se. As discussed in Chapter 1, for patients with diabetes, ACE inhibitors and angiotensin receptor blockers (ARBs) reduce albuminuria and may offer reno-protection independent of their BP-lowering effects[31,32] and are therefore the preferred first-line agents in our protocols outlined below. This recommendation differs slightly from the current ADA recommendation that ACE inhibitors or ARBs (but not both together), thiazide-like diuretics, or dihydropyridine calcium channel blockers, which have all been shown to reduce ASCVD in patients with diabetes, may be used for treating hypertension (although the ADA still recommends an ACE inhibitor or an ARB as the initial drug in patients with albuminuria).

The efficacy of anti-hypertension agents may also be more pronounced if dosed in the evening. A meta-analysis of trials comparing monotherapy administered in the evening or the morning found better overall 24-hour BP control with bedtime dosing.[33] Another prospective, comparative trial, specifically in hypertensive individuals with diabetes found that administration of at least one anti-hypertension agent at bedtime led to not only better overall BP control, but also significantly fewer ASCVD events after 5.4 years of follow-up, compared to all agents taken only in the morning.[34] However, most patients are still accustomed to dosing their medications in the morning. Thus, our treatment algorithm (below) recommends taking advantage of evening dosing when doses are escalated (i.e., split to b.i.d.), rather than simply increasing the single morning dose.

Each class of anti-hypertension agents is discussed below in greater detail, and all agents currently approved by the U.S. Food and Drug Administration (FDA) for hypertension treatment are listed in Table 5.1. The ADA recommends that, after lifestyle modification and the appropriate use of ACE inhibitors or ARBs to both control BP and provide reno-protection, selected diuretic and calcium channel blocker agents may be added if BP targets have not been achieved.[16] Our algorithm, however, recommends a more specific sequence of medication choices, titrated according to a specific protocol. So while our protocol differs from the ADA recommendations, they are still consistent with the same underlying treatment principles and aim to achieve the same therapeutic goals. Although the combination agents also listed in Table 5.1 are not used in our treatment algorithm, they may still be used to simplify medication regimens, if available, once the patient's anti-hypertension medication requirements to achieve their BP goal using a stepped-care approach have been established.

ACE INHIBITORS

The renin-angiotensin-aldosterone system (RAAS) is a major regulator of body hemodynamics,[35] as depicted in Fig. 5.1. ACE inhibitors interrupt the conversion of angiotensin I into active angiotensin II, which is a potent vasoconstrictor. Angiotensin II, in turn, activates the angiotensin (AT_1) receptor, leading to production of aldosterone, a mineralocorticoid that contributes to renal sodium reabsorption at

Table 5.1. Anti-Hypertension Medications

Generic name	Brand name(s)	Starting daily dose	Maximum daily dose
ACE inhibitors			
Benazepril	Lotensin	10 mg (q.d. or b.i.d.)	80 mg/day[a]
Captopril	Capoten	12.5–25 mg (b.i.d. or t.i.d.)	450 mg/day
Enalapril	Vasotec, Epaned	5 mg (q.d. or b.i.d.)	40 mg/day
Fosinopril	Monopril	10 mg q.d.	80 mg q.d.
Lisinopril	Prinivil, Zestril	10 mg q.d.	80 mg q.d.
Moexipril	Univasc	7.5 mg q.d.	30 mg q.d.
Perindopril	Aceon	4 mg (q.d. or b.i.d.)	16 mg/day
Quinapril	Accupril	10 mg q.d.	80 mg q.d.
Ramipril	Altace	2.5 mg (q.d. or b.i.d.)	20 mg/day
Trandolapril	Mavik	1–2 mg q.d.	8 mg q.d.
Angiotensin receptor blockers (ARBs)			
Azilsartan	Edarbi	80 mg q.d.	80 mg q.d.
Candesartan	Atacand	16 mg (q.d. or b.i.d.)	32 mg/day
Eprosartan	Teveten	600 mg (q.d. or b.i.d.)	800 mg/day
Irbesartan	Avapro	150 mg q.d.	300 mg q.d.
Losartan	Cozaar	50 mg (q.d. or b.i.d.)	100 mg/day
Olmesartan	Benicar	20 mg q.d.	40 mg q.d.
Telmisartan	Micardis	40 mg q.d.	160 mg q.d.
Valsartan	Diovan	80 mg q.d.	320 mg q.d.
Thiazide diuretics			
Chlorothiazide	Diuril	250 mg (q.d. or b.i.d.)	2,000 mg/day
Chlorthalidone	Thalitone	12.5–25 mg q.d.	50 mg q.d.
Hydrochlorothiazide	Microzide	12.5–50 mg q.d.	50 mg q.d.[b]
Indapamide	Lozol	1.25 mg q.a.m.	5 mg q.d.[c]
Methychlothiazide	Aquatensen	2.5 mg q.d.	5 mg q.d.
Metolazone	Zaroxolyn	2.5 mg q.d.	5 mg q.d.
Loop diuretics			
Bumetanide	Bumex	0.5 mg (q.d. or b.i.d.)	10 mg/day
Ethacrynic acid	Edecrin	25 mg (q.d. or b.i.d. or t.i.d.)	100 mg/day
Furosemide	Lasix	10–40 mg b.i.d.	600 mg/day
Torsemide	Demadex	5 mg q.d.	10 mg q.d.
CCBs			

(continued on page 128)

Table 5.1. Anti-Hypertension Medications *(continued)*

Generic name	Brand name(s)	Starting daily dose	Maximum daily dose
Amlodipine	Norvasc	5 mg q.d.	10 mg q.d.
Diltiazem ER (12-hour)	Cardizem SR	60–120 mg b.i.d.	360 mg/day
Diltiazem ER (24-hour)	Cardizem CD Cardizem LA Cartia XT Dilacor XR Dilt-CD Diltia XT Taztia XT Tiazac	120–240 mg q.d.	48–540 mg/day[d]
Felodipine	Plendil	5 mg q.d.	10 mg q.d.
Isradipine	Dynacirc CR	2.5 mg b.i.d.	10 mg/day
Nifedipine ER	Adalat CC Afeditab CR Nifediac CC Nifedical XL Procardia XL	30 mg q.d.	90–120 mg/day
Nicardipine	Cardene	20 mg t.i.d.	120 mg/day
	Cardene SR	30 mg b.i.d.	120 mg/day
Nisoldipine ER	Sular	17–20 mg q.d.	34–60 mg q.d.
Verapamil (immediate-release)	Calan	80 mg t.i.d.	480 mg/day
Verapamil ER (12-hour)	Calan SR	180 mg (q.a.m. or b.i.d.)	480 mg/day
Verapamil ER (24-hour AM)	Verelan	240 mg q.a.m.	480 mg/day
Verapamil ER (24-hour PM)	Verelan PM	200 mg q.h.s.	400 mg/day
Direct vasodilators			
Hydralazine	Apresoline	10–25 mg q.i.d.	300 mg/day[e]
Minoxidil	Loniten	5 mg (q.d. or b.i.d.)	100 mg/day
β-Adrenergic receptor antagonists (β-blockers)			
Acebutolol	Sectral	400 mg q.d.	1,200 mg q.d.
Atenolol	Tenormin	50 mg q.d.	100 mg q.d.
Betaxolol	Kerlone	10 mg q.d.	40 mg q.d.
Bisoprolol	Zebeta	5 mg q.d.	20 mg q.d.
Carvedilol	Coreg	6.25 mg b.i.d.	50 mg/day
Carvedilol ER	Coreg CR	20 mg q.d.	80 mg q.d.
Labetalol	Trandate	100 mg b.i.d.	2,400 mg/day

Generic name	Brand name(s)	Starting daily dose	Maximum daily dose
Metoprolol	Lopressor	50 mg b.i.d.	450 mg/day
Metoprolol ER	Toprol XL	25 mg q.d.	400 mg q.d.
Nadolol	Corgard	40 mg q.d.	320 mg q.d.
Nebivolol	Bystolic	5 mg q.d.	40 mg q.d.
Penbutolol	Levatol	20 mg q.d.	80 mg q.d.
Pindolol	Visken	5 mg b.i.d.	60 mg/day
Propranolol	Inderal	40 mg b.i.d.	640 mg/day
Propranolol ER	Inderal LA InnoPran XL	80 mg q.d.	120–640 mg q.d.
Timolol	Blocadren	10 mg b.i.d.	60 mg/day
Aldosterone receptor antagonists (potassium-sparing diuretics)			
Amiloride	Midamor	5 mg q.d.	20 mg q.d.
Eplerenone	Inspra	50 mg (q.d. or b.i.d.)	100 mg/day
Spironolactone	Aldactone	12.5 mg (q.d. or b.i.d.)	50 mg/day
Direct renin inhibitor			
Aliskiren	Tekturna	150 mg q.d.	300 mg q.d.
α-Adrenergic receptor agonists (central and peripheral sympatholytics)			
Clonidine	Catapres	0.1 mg b.i.d.	2.4 mg/day
Clonidine ER	Nexiclon XR	0.17 mg q.h.s.	0.52 mg/day
Clonidine Transdermal	Catapres TTS	0.1 mg/24-hour patch, apply once each week	0.6 mg/24-hour patch, apply once each week
Guanfacine	Tenex	1 mg q.h.s.	3 mg q.h.s.
Methyldopa	Aldomet	250 mg (b.i.d. or t.i.d.)	3,000 mg/day
Reserpine	(generic only)	0.5 mg q.d. load, then 0.05–0.1 mg q.d.	0.5 mg q.d.
α-Adrenergic receptor antagonists (α-blockers)			
Doxazosin	Cardura	1 mg q.d.	16 mg q.d.
Prazosin	Minipress	1 mg (b.i.d. or t.i.d.)	20 mg/day
Terazosin	Hytrin	1 mg (q.h.s. or b.i.d.)	20 mg/day
Combination agents			

(continued on page 130)

Table 5.1. Anti-Hypertension Medications *(continued)*

Generic name	Brand name(s)	Starting daily dose	Maximum daily dose
Benazepril/ hydrochlorothiazide	Lotensin HCT	5/6.25 mg q.d.	20/25 mg q.d.
Captopril/ hydrochlorothiazide	Capozide	25/15 mg (q.d. or b.i.d. or t.i.d.)	150/50 mg/day
Enalapril/ hydrochlorothiazide	Vaseretic	5/12.5 mg q.d.	20/50 mg q.d.
Fosinopril/ hydrochlorothiazide	Monopril-HCT	10/12.5 mg q.d.	20/12.5 mg q.d.
Lisinopril/ hydrochlorothiazide	Prinzide Zestoretic	10/12.5 mg q.d.	40/50 mg q.d.
Moexipril/ hydrochlorothiazide	Uniretic	7.5/12.5 mg (q.d. or b.i.d.)	30/50 mg/day
Quinapril/ hydrochlorothiazide	Accuretic	10/12.5 mg q.d.	20/25 mg q.d.
Azilsartan/ chlorthalidone	Edarbyclor	40/12.5 mg q.d.	40/25 mg q.d.
Candesartan/ hydrochlorothiazide	Atacand HCT	16/12.5 mg (q.d. or b.i.d.)	32/25 mg/day
Eprosartan/ hydrochlorothiazide	Teveten HCT	600/12.5 mg q.d.	600/25 mg q.d.
Irbesartan/ hydrochlorothiazide	Avalide	150/12.5 mg q.d.	300/25 mg q.d.
Losartan/ hydrochlorothiazide	Hyzaar	50/12.5 mg q.d.	100/25 mg q.d.
Olmesartan/ hydrochlorothiazide	Benicar HCT	20/12.5 mg q.d.	40/25 mg q.d.
Telmisartan/ hydrochlorothiazide	Micardis HCT	40/12.5 mg q.d.	160/25 mg q.d.
Valsartan/ hydrochlorothiazide	Diovan HCT	160/12.5 mg q.d.	320/25 mg q.d.
Amlodipine/benazepril	Lotrel	2.5/10 mg q.d.	10/40 mg q.d.
Perindopril/amlodipine	Prestalia	3.5/2.5 mg q.d.	14/10 mg q.d.
Trandolapril/ verapamil ER	Tarka	1/240 mg q.d.	8/480 mg q.d.
Amlodipine/ olmesartan	Azor	5/20 mg q.d.	10/40 mg q.d.
Telmisartan/ amlodipine	Twynsta	40/5 mg q.d.	80/10 mg q.d.
Amlodipine/valsartan	Exforge	5/160 mg q.d.	10/320 mg q.d.
Olmesartan/ amlodipine/ hydrochlorothiazide	Tribenzor	20/5/12.5 mg q.d.	40/10/25 mg q.d.

Generic name	Brand name(s)	Starting daily dose	Maximum daily dose
Amlodipine/valsartan/ hydrochlorothiazide	Exforge HCT	5/160/12.5 mg q.d.	10/320/25 mg q.d.
Atenolol/ chlorthalidone	Tenoretic	50/25 mg q.d.	100/25 mg q.d.
Bisoprolol/ hydrochlorothiazide	Ziac	2.5/6.25 mg q.d.	10/6.25 mg q.d.
Metoprolol/ hydrochlorothiazide	Lopressor HCT	50/25 mg (q.d. or b.i.d.)	200/50 mg/day
Metoprolol ER/ hydrochlorothiazide	Dutoprol	25/12.5 mg q.d.	200/25 mg q.d.
Nadolol/ bendroflumethiazide	Corzide	40/5 mg q.d.	80/5 mg q.d.
Propranolol/ hydrochlorothiazide	(generic only)	40/25 mg b.i.d.	160/50 mg/day
Amiloride/ hydrochlorothiazide	(generic only)	5/50 mg q.d.	10/100 mg q.d.
Spironolactone/ hydrochlorothiazide	Aldactazide	12.5/12.5 mg (q.d. or b.i.d.)	200/200 mg/day
Triamterene/ hydrochlorothiazide	Dyazide Maxzide	37.5/25 mg q.d.	75/50 mg q.d.
Aliskiren/ hydrochlorothiazide	Tekturna HCT	150/12.5 mg q.d.	300/25 mg q.d.
Aliskiren/amlodipine	Tekamlo	150/5 mg q.d.	300/10 mg q.d.
Aliskiren/amlodipine/ hydrochlorothiazide	Amturnide	150/5/12.5 mg q.d.	300/10/25 mg q.d.
Clonidine/ chlorthalidone	Clorpres	0.1/15 mg (q.d. or b.i.d.)	0.6/30 mg/day

Because the incremental BP-lowering benefit of anti-hypertension agents is less at the upper limits of the dose range, our algorithm outlined below limits the maximum daily doses to [a]40 mg for benazepril, [b]25 mg for hydrochlorothiazide, [c]2.5 mg for indapamide, [d]360 mg for diltiazem extended release (ER), and [e]200 mg for hydralazine.

the distal tubule. Thus, ACE inhibitors reduce BP by reducing both angiotensin II action on the vasculature and aldosterone-mediated sodium reabsorption. In addition, they provide proven survival benefits when used in post–myocardial infarction patients with severe heart failure or left ventricular dysfunction.[36] As anti-hypertension agents, they are supported by many studies that collectively show impressive reductions in ASCVD and all-cause mortality.[37,38]

An important side effect of ACE inhibitors is hyperkalemia, which is more likely to occur in patients with some preexisting renal insufficiency, so in such patients, serum potassium levels should be monitored more closely. Between 10 and 40% of patients may also develop a persistent (yet non-serious) non-productive cough, which usually requires switching to an alternate agent (usually an ARB). In patients with renal artery stenosis or relative dehydration (e.g., concomitant diuretic use) wherein maintenance of glomerular filtration depends on intra-glomerular vasoconstriction of the efferent arteriole, ACE inhibitors may cause a fall in GFR or mild hypotension, so in such cases, estimated glomerular filtration rates (eGFRs) and/or the patient's clinical response should be monitored more closely. A rare, but potentially life-threatening idiosyncratic reaction is angioedema, manifesting as swelling of the lips, mouth, tongue, and throat; it occurs only in 1 to 2 individuals per 1,000 individuals (but possibly higher among African-American patients), and in such cases, the ACE inhibitor should be promptly discontinued and switched to an ARB. ACE inhibitors are also contraindicated in pregnancy because of adverse fetal effects in the second and third trimesters.[36] As a general rule, African-American patients tend to respond relatively less effectively to ACE inhibitors than compared to patients of other races, so slightly higher doses may be needed to achieve the same effect.[39] However, this subtle racial difference in BP response is abolished when a thiazide diuretic or a calcium channel blocker is added to the ACE inhibitor.[40]

ANGIOTENSIN RECEPTOR BLOCKERS (ARBs)

ARBs competitively inhibit the binding of angiotensin II to the angiotensin receptor, thereby also reducing both the vasoconstriction of angiotensin II and sodium retention through reducing aldosterone secretion[41] (Figure 5.1). In many ways, their effectiveness in patients with diabetes is equivalent to that of ACE inhibitors, although ARBs are more expensive. However, recent meta-analyses found that the evidence basis for reducing ASCVD events and mortality as anti-hypertension agents was not as strong with ARBs compared to ACE inhibitors.[37,38,42] As with ACE inhibitors, hyperkalemia remains a potential concern, particularly in patients with preexisting renal insufficiency. Also, declining renal function with ARB treatment remains a potential concern in patients with renal artery stenosis. However, unlike ACE inhibitors, ARBs are not associated with a dry cough, and there is less risk of angioedema. And as with the ACE inhibitors, African-American patients may respond less well, necessitating slightly higher doses, and ARBs are also contraindicated in pregnancy.[41] Studies examining the combined use of ACE inhibitors and ARBs together have generally failed to show any additive benefits, while problems such as hyperkalemia can be magnified, so the combined use of both classes is not recommended.[43]

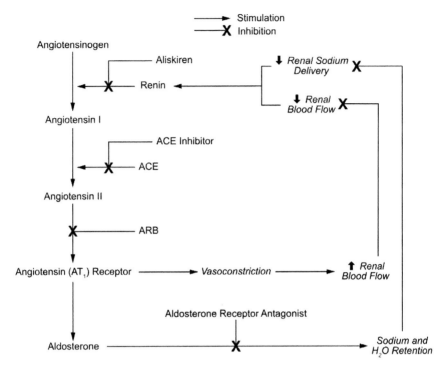

Figure 5.1. The renin-angiotensin-aldosterone system.

THIAZIDE AND LOOP DIURETICS

Thiazide diuretics principally inhibit sodium reabsorption at the distal renal tubules, thus increasing urinary sodium excretion and reducing the extracellular fluid volume, but they also possess vasodilatory properties through both direct and indirect mechanisms, as well as reduce BP through other potential mechanisms.[44] And because sodium retention is a manifestation of insulin resistance and hyperinsulinemia,[45] a diuretic is often an effective option for patients with diabetes.

The ALLHAT study, which included a subset of patients with diabetes, actually found that, although reduction of the primary outcome of all composite ASCVD events was similar for several different anti-hypertension agents, chlorthalidone was superior to amlodipine for reducing heart failure and was actually superior to lisinopril for reducing combined ASCVD events, strokes, and heart failure.[46] In the Seventh Report of the Joint National Committee on Prevention, Detection, Evaluation, and Treatment of High Blood Pressure (JNC 7),[47] thiazides were recommended as a first-line choice for the general population with uncomplicated hypertension (based largely on overall equivalent benefit together with good tolerability and lower cost), while for patients with chronic renal disease (including indidivuals with diabetic kidney disease), they remain an ideal second-line agent following the first-line use of ACE inhibitors or ARBs (and they may also help to offset the risk of hyperkalemia with ACE inhibitor or ARB mono-therapy). The updated 2014 JNC guidelines (JNC 8)[48] preserved the recommendation for ACE inhibitors or ARBs as the preferred treatment in patients with nephropathy. JNC 8 also recommended that for African-American patients in the general population, thiazide diuretics (or calcium channel blockers [see below]) may be a preferred first-line choice,[48] based on findings from ALLHAT showing that in the African-American subgroup, chlorthalidone was superior to lisinopril for reducing strokes and combined ASCVD.[46] However, the ADA recommendations for diabetes patients[16] have consistently emphasized the use of ACE inhibitors or ARBs as an important medication choice for the anti-hypertension agent regimen for all diabetes patients, regardless of race (and with thiazide diuretics as a reasonable second, add-on choice).

Thiazide diuretics are generally well tolerated. Increased potassium loss occurs mostly within the first week of therapy, and with the lower dosages used today, overall reductions in serum potassium levels are usually minor and treatable with addition of triamterene or potassium supplements. Effects of thiazides on worsening insulin resistance remain unresolved; among nondiabetic individuals they have traditionally been associated with a greater risk of new-onset diabetes (possibly related to their potassium-lowering actions influencing insulin production[49]). It is generally believed that most thiazides are less effective in the presence of renal insufficiency and should not be used if eGFR is <30 mL/min, but indapamide and metolazone may retain their effects better at lower GFR levels. Thiazide diuretics may also cause slight increases in calcium and uric acid, but these increases are rarely of any clinical significance[50] (except that it may indicate early primary hyperparathyroidism[51]). Diuretics may also increase total cholesterol dose-dependently, particularly among African-Americans, as well as increased triglycerides and reduced HDL cholesterol, specifically in patients with kidney disease attributed to diabetes.[52] Also, because thiazides contain sulfur, they should be used with caution in patients with severe allergies to sulfa-containing medications.

Loop diuretics also inhibit renal sodium reabsorption at the distal tubules, but also within the ascending loop of Henle, producing a more profound diuresis than thiazides; unlike thiazides, they produce much less peripheral vasodilation.[53] They tend to be short-acting agents (with the exception of torsemide), so aside from multiple-daily dosing, the compensatory RAAS activation in response to volume depletion makes them less effective anti-hypertension agents overall; they are more often used in fluid overload states such as peripheral edema or heart failure. One meta-analysis of loop diuretic trials found only a modest overall lowering of BP.[54] Studies directly comparing loop diuretics to thiazides are small and poorly designed,[53] and there are no outcome studies supporting their efficacy for ASCVD or renal outcomes, so they should not be used as first-line choices. However, they may serve as an adjunct to other agents in states of volume overload, and because they may retain their effect at very low GFR levels (<30 mL/min) better than thiazides, they may have a role for BP control in severe renal insufficiency[16] (although higher doses are still required as GFR continues to fall). Potential side effects are similar to those of thiazide diuretics, except that they may cause calcium wasting rather than retention. For patients with severe allergies to sulfa-containing medications, ethacrynic acid represents a safe alternative.[53]

CALCIUM CHANNEL BLOCKERS

Calcium channel blockers (CCBs) may cause arteriolar dilation, thus reducing peripheral vascular resistance, as well as reduce cardiac contractility and slow cardiac conduction so as to reduce cardiac output. There are two broad classes of CCBs: non-dihydropyridine (NDHP) CCBs (diltiazem, verapamil), which are more selective for the direct cardiac effects than the peripheral vasculature, and dihydropyridine (DHP) CCBs (amlodipine, felodipine, isradipine, nifedipine, nicardipine, nisoldipine), which are more selective for the peripheral vasculature than the direct cardiac effects.[55] Thus, NDHP CCBs are more likely to predispose to heart block and bradyarrhythmias in susceptible individuals (such as with concurrent use of certain β-adrenergic antagonists), while DHP CCBs are more likely to predispose to peripheral edema, reflex sympathetic tachycardia, headaches, and flushing. In general, adverse effects are lower with the more extended-release formulations that are more commonly used today.

Many head-to-head comparison studies of CCBs versus other agents, and meta-analyses of such comparison studies, have generally found that CCBs may be inferior to ACE inhibitors and/or diuretics for a variety of ASCVD outcome measures in patients with diabetes,[56-58] although not in all such analyses.[59] Similar findings have been seen with studies in the general population,[60] along with some analyses suggesting that CCBs may also be superior to β-adrenergic antagonists.[61,62] In some cases, African-American patients in the general population may respond to CCBs more consistently than with other agents,[63] with slightly greater BP lowering compared to white patients,[64] or with greater reduction of strokes,[65] but the actual BP differences are subtle. JNC 8 recommends that for African-Americans in the general population, a CCB (or a thiazide diuretic) may be a preferred first-line choice (and JNC 8 extrapolates that recommendation to African-Americans with diabetes, since 46% of African-American participants in ALLHAT also had diabetes[48]). However, the ADA recommendations do not make such a distinction with respect to the role of CCBs in African-Americans with diabetes and instead still emphasize the preferred use of ACE inhibitors or ARBs as first-line choices for all patients with diabetes.[16]

In terms of effects on renal function in patients with kidney disease attributed to diabetes, some head-to-head comparative studies have shown that the albuminuria reduction and/or preservation of GFR with nifedipine[66] and amlodipine[67] was comparable to that of ACE inhibitors (the effect being largely a function of the degree of BP lowering). However, other studies have shown differential effects, with the CCB (nifedipine) being inferior to the ACE inhibitor after 1 year,[68] and with differences sustained at a 5.5-year observational follow-up.[69] Even among CCBs, the different mechanisms of action between DHP and NDHP CCBs may differentially affect diabetic kidney disease. DHP CCBs more preferentially vasodilate glomerular afferent arterioles, leading to glomerular hyperfiltration and possible scarring, in comparison to NDHP CCBs. Thus, DHP CCBs may not reduce (or may increase) proteinuria, whereas NDHP CCBs more consistently reduce proteinuria and may slow the loss of glomerular function.[70,71] Given that albuminuria is an important marker of diabetic kidney disease, it follows that NDHP CCBs might be the preferred choice of CCB in patients with diabetes. However, the clinical significance of this difference for long-term preservation of renal function in diabetes remains unclear, with at least one comparison trial finding no significant difference between verapamil SR and amlodipine when used with ACE inhibitors in diabetic nephropathy patients.[72] Thus, in our treatment algorithm (below), ACE inhibitors or ARBs remain as the first-line anti-hypertension agent choice and diuretics are still the second-line choice, but a NDHP CCB serves as the preferred third-line choice.

DIRECT VASODILATORS

These agents directly act on vascular smooth muscle cells to cause vasodilation. As monotherapy, patients rapidly develop tolerance to these agents as a result of reflex increases in sympathetic activity and activation of the RAAS. Therefore, ideally, they should be avoided in patients with ischemic cardiac disease or heart failure, and they should only be used in combination with other anti-hypertension agent classes. In our algorithms presented below, they serve as a fourth-line drug choice.

Hydralazine causes arterial vasodilation through a nitric oxide–dependent pathway. It is inactivated by the genetically determined trait of acetylation; about half of the U.S. population are "slow acetylators" who metabolize hydralazine more slowly. Therefore, these individuals may not only have enhanced anti-hypertension effects, but are also more likely to experience side effects, including headaches, nasal congestion, peripheral edema, gastrointestinal intolerance, peripheral neuropathy (due to pyridoxine deficiency), and, at high doses (>200 mg/day), leucopenia and/or a drug-induced lupus-like syndrome (which is discernible from classic systemic lupus erythematosis by serological testing of single-stranded DNA instead of double-stranded DNA). However, when used in combination with other anti-hypertension agents, the adverse effect of the "slow acetylator" phenotype may not affect the therapeutic response.[73]

Minoxidil causes peripheral vasodilation through activation of potassium channels in vascular smooth muscle, but it produces a hemodynamic effect similar to hydralazine. As such, it can also cause headaches, nasal congestion, and peripheral edema. However, minoxidil does not cause a drug-induced lupus-like syndrome, although it does cause reversible hypertrichosis, which can limit its use, particularly in women. Pericardial and pleural effusions may also occur idiosyncratically.[74] No studies exist to support its ASCVD benefits as an anti-hypertension agent. Because of the side effects of minoxidil, it is now used only in truly refractory cases of hypertension, particularly in patients with chronic kidney disease.

β-ADRENERGIC RECEPTOR ANTAGONISTS (β-BLOCKERS)

Antagonism of β-adrenergic receptors produces multiple and varied vasoactive effects, depending on the selectivity of the β-adrenergic receptor subtypes being blocked. β_1-Adrenergic receptors principally increase cardiac contractility and impulse conduction, so selective β_1-blockers (e.g., acebutolol, atenolol, betaxolol, bisoprolol, metoprolol, and nebivolol) principally reduce heart rate and cardiac output ("cardioselectivity"). β_2-Adrenergic receptors principally increase pulmonary bronchodilation and peripheral vascular relaxation, so β_2 blockade may exacerbate reactive airways and precipitate peripheral vasoconstriction. Nonselective β-blockers (e.g., carvedilol, nadolol, propranolol, and timolol) will have mixed effects on both receptor subtypes; at high doses, even a selective β-blocker may have crossover effects on other receptor subtypes. These agents can also differ according to intrinsic sympathomimetic activity (ISA), or partial agonist effects on β-adrenergic receptors (e.g., acebutolol, labetolol, penbutolol, and pindolol), which are less likely to cause excessive bradycardia. Some agents also possess α_1-antagonist effects (e.g., carvedilol and labetalol), leading to additional peripheral vasodilatory effects. Nebivolol additionally acts on nitric oxide to provide further vasodilation.

For the general population and for patients with diabetes, β-blockers have been proven to be cardio-protective in the post–myocardial infarction setting by virtue of reducing myocardial oxygen demand,[75-77] and for heart failure patients by virtue of their negative effects on cardiac contractility,[77,78] in addition to being anti-hypertension agents.[79] Early outcome studies of their use for hypertension, such as the UKPDS in patients with diabetes, actually showed that β-blockers (atenolol) not only reduced BP comparably to an ACE inhibitor (captopril), but that they reduced macrovascular, microvascular, and renal end points to a similar extent.[80] However, the Losartan Intervention for Endpoint Reduction in Hypertension (LIFE) study found that among somewhat older individuals with diabetes, atenolol was inferior to an ARB (losartan) for reducing ASCVD events, ASCVD deaths, and all-cause mortality, despite comparable BP lowering.[81] Thus, while β-blockers can be effective anti-hypertension agents, they may not be uniformly effective for all patients with diabetes. Various meta-analyses have come to mixed conclusions about the wisdom of using β-blockers as early anti-hypertension agent choices for the general population, with some showing benefits comparable to other classes of agents, while others showing inferiority with respect to ASCVD, strokes, and mortality outcomes (and only marginally better than placebo).[82]

Older agents such as atenolol or metoprolol have also been associated with increased glucose levels, worsened insulin resistance, and/or adverse lipid profiles,[83,84] consistent with a general observation across many trials that these older β-blockers may precipitate more new-onset diabetes among nondiabetic participants than agents of other classes.[82] A reduction in metabolic activity and energy consumption is believed to account for a small weight gain that may be seen with β-blocker use.[85] Older β-blockers may slightly raise triglyceride levels, although cardioselective agents with ISA may slightly lower cholesterol levels.[52] The Glycemic Effects in Diabetes Mellitus: Carvedilol–Metoprolol Comparison in Hypertensives (GEMINI) trial found that carvedilol significantly improved A1C and insulin sensitivity compared to metoprolol and also led to less weight gain and less progression to microalbuminuria, despite comparable BP lowering.[86,87] In general, agents with peripheral vasodilatory properties (e.g., carvedilol, labetalol, and nebivolol) tend to have more favorable metabolic effects than those without vasodilatory properties.[88] Thus, while they may still be beneficial for BP lowering, most β-blockers (except perhaps carvedilol) should not be early anti-hypertension agent choices. The JNC 8 recommendations do not support the use of β-blockers as a first-line choice.[48]

In general, β-blockers will reduce exercise tolerance, by virtue of their negative actions on the entire cardiovascular system,[77] making them less ideal for younger, active individuals. And as with ACE inhibitors and ARBs, African-American patients may respond to β-blockers slightly less effectively than others, although this may not translate into differences in clinical outcomes.[63] β-Blockers may also be associated with a variety of other undesirable side effects, including somnolence, lethargy, depression, blurred vision, and sleep disturbances.[77] Cardioselective β-blockers should still be used with caution in patients with significant asthma or chronic obstructive pulmonary disease, or peripheral vascular conditions such as Raynaud's phenomenon, peripheral arterial disease, or erectile dysfunction, because of potential crossover β_2-antagonism. Their negative effects on cardiac conduction, particularly the agents without ISA, may worsen heart block or other bradyarrhythmias in predisposed individuals (such as those concurrently using other agents that slow cardiac conduction, like NDHP CCBs). While the survival benefits of β-blockers for post–myocardial infarction patients are clear, abrupt discontinuation can precipitate angina; any withdrawal should instead be a slow taper of the dose. And while it is commonly believed that β-blockers in patients with diabetes may blunt the symptoms of hypoglycemia and/or slow the recovery from a hypoglycemic episode, there is actually little clinical evidence that such phenomena actually occur.

ALDOSTERONE RECEPTOR ANTAGONISTS (POTASSIUM-SPARING DIURETICS)

Aldosterone acts principally at the distal renal tubules and collecting ducts to promote sodium reabsorption and potassium excretion, so aldosterone antagonists lower BP by principally enhancing sodium excretion (Figure 5.1). Amiloride is an older, noncompetitive potassium sparing agent[89] that is now largely only used together with other diuretics. The nonselective, competitive aldosterone antagonist, spironolactone, has been shown to improve survival in severe heart failure[90] as well as improve BP control for the general population when used as a third-line agent on top of background therapy that includes ACE inhibitors.[91] However, it has not been shown to reduce ASCVD outcomes as an anti-hypertension agent, and hyperkalemia remains a concern whenever these agents are added to ACE inhibitors or ARBs, so regular monitoring of potassium levels is recommended within 2–4 weeks of initiation or dose increase. Spironolactone also antagonizes progesterone and androgen receptors, leading to menstrual abnormalities in premenopausal women and gynecomastia and erectile dysfunction in men.[91] Eplerenone is a more selective aldosterone antagonist and does not cause these same side effects. It has also been shown to improve survival for patients with heart failure.[92] Good quality studies of the efficacy of aldosterone antagonists in diabetic patients with chronic renal insufficiency are limited. Meta-analyses that included diabetic patients have found that aldosterone antagonists, when added to ACE inhibitors or ARBs, further improve BP and proteinuria, but fail to improve GFR, and yet cause a substantial increase in hyperkalemia,[93,94] particularly among older patients with more longstanding diabetes or those with preexisting renal insufficiency or hyperkalemia.

DIRECT RENIN INHIBITORS

In the RAAS, renin is secreted by the renal juxtaglomerular apparatus in response to perceived volume depletion and converts inactive angiotensinogen to angiotensin I (the precursor of angiotensin II that is acted upon by ACE; see Figure 5.1). Currently, aliskiren is the only FDA-approved drug in this class of direct renin inhibitors. As monotherapy, it generally lowers BP as effectively as other agents; is longer-acting (terminal half-life of 40 hours), which produces sustained BP benefits over at least 24 hours; and is generally well tolerated.[95] Uncommon side effects include hypotension (particularly with preexisting volume depletion) and peripheral edema; cough occurs less commonly than with ACE inhibitors, and angioedema is rare. As with ACE inhibitors and ARBs, aliskiren should be avoided in cases of pregnancy and bilateral renal artery stenosis. Hyperkalemia occurs uncommonly when used as monotherapy, but the risk increases substantially if it is used concurrently with ACE inhibitors or ARBs. However, BP lowering may be additive when it is combined with diuretics or CCBs.[95] Not unexpectedly, aliskiren has been shown to reduce albuminuria when added to background anti-hypertension treatment in patients with diabetes, independent of BP changes.[96] However, when used together with ACE inhibitors or ARBs in high-risk individuals with diabetes with eGFR <60 mL/min, there was a significant increase in the incidence of nonfatal strokes, worsening renal dysfunction, hyperkalemia, and hypotension, along with no detectable ASCVD benefit.[97] Thus, given that ACE inhibitors or ARBs are widely used as first-line therapy, addition of aliskiren in such diabetes patients is not recommended,[95] just as combined use of ACE inhibitors plus ARBs is not recommended.

α_2-ADRENERGIC RECEPTOR AGONISTS (CENTRAL AND PERIPHERAL SYMPATHOLYTICS)

Activation of central presynaptic α_2-adrenergic receptors in the brainstem reduces sympathetic activity at the heart and/or peripheral vasculature; methyldopa, clonidine, and guanfacine are currently available central sympatholytic agents approved for the treatment of hypertension in the U.S. There are no good quality studies of these agents showing ASCVD event reductions in patients with hypertension. As a group, they are often associated with side effects such as dry mouth, fatigue, or somnolence, and short-acting formulations may be prone to rebound hypertension if dosed intermittently; sustained dosing is required to be effective.[98] They should also be used with caution with β-blockers because of their synergistic effects to induce bradycardia. Methyldopa predominantly reduces peripheral vascular resistance and is now used most commonly in pregnancy because of low teratogenicity, but it may also be associated with hypersensitivity reactions, including hepatitis, Coombs-positive hemolytic anemia, gynecomastia, and Parkinson's exacerbation. Clonidine predominantly reduces cardiac output, but the short-acting oral formulation is particularly prone to rebound hypertension if not dosed at least twice a day; a longer-acting transdermal system produces more gradual and sustained effects, although local skin reactions may occur and require treatment with hydrocortisone cream. Guanfacine acts mainly on the peripheral vasculature, has a longer half-life than the other agents, and may be associated with less rebound hypertension.[98]

Peripheral sympatholytics deplete norepinephrine from the post-ganglionic sympathetic nerves, which reduces cardiac and neurogenic vascular tone. Reserpine is predominantly a peripheral sympatholytic,[98] but is rarely used today because of multiple side effects such as nasal congestion, depression and suicide risk, increased gastric acidity and other gastrointestinal intolerances, orthostatic hypotension, erectile dysfunction, and fatigue and somnolence. Although reserpine effectively lowers systolic BP, studies on its efficacy are limited.[99]

α_1-ADRENERGIC RECEPTOR ANTAGONISTS (α-BLOCKERS)

α_1-Adrenergic receptors, located predominantly on vascular smooth muscle cells, mediate the vasoconstrictive action of norepinephrine. The pivotal ALLHAT study, a head-to-head comparison of various anti-hypertension agent classes, found the α-blocker doxazosin to be inferior for ASCVD event reduction,[30] substantially reducing the use of these agents for hypertension. However, α_1-adrenergic receptors also regulate the constriction of urinary sphincters, so these agents actually have greater utility for the treatment of urinary hesitancy in benign prostatic hypertrophy.[100] A recent meta-analysis of α-blocker agents confirmed that the anti-hypertension efficacy of these agents, while measurable, remains modest at best.[101] Side effects of α-blockers are generally minimal, except for potential "first-dose" orthostatic hypotension, which occurs with initial exposure to the drug, but usually wanes with continued therapy as renal hemodynamics compensate. Thus, treatment should begin at the lowest dose,[100] ideally taken at bedtime.

Thus, with so many choices of anti-hypertension agents available, a simplified treatment algorithm that applies many of the evidence-based rationales discussed above will be a useful guide for clinicians treating hypertensive diabetes patients. Outlined below is the algorithm that we use at our institution.

HYPERTENSION ALGORITHM

Our algorithm below may differ from the recommendations of the ADA. Specific drug choices within this algorithm are limited to those available at our institution. While different agents may be available at other institutions and may be substituted within the same medication class, we still recommend using these same classes of drugs in the sequence presented below.

1. Initial hypertension treatment is medical nutritional therapy (MNT) and lifestyle modification. If BP is ≥140/90 mmHg (when repeated), start pharmacological treatment.
2. Principles of treatment to achieve the BP goal of <140/90 mmHg:
   a) To determine the effect of starting or changing the dose of an anti-hypertension medication, measure the BP approximately 4 weeks after initiating or changing the dose.

b) If BP goal of <140/90 mmHg is not reached at the maximum (tolerated) dose of a class of drugs, add the drug from the next class.

c) To the extent possible, some doses of anti-hypertension medications should be given in the evening (i.e., twice a day), with the exception of diuretics.

A. Nonpharmacological therapy (lifestyle change)

- Weight reduction of at least 5–10% of initial weight if overweight or obese
- Sodium restriction to <2,300 mg/day, along with increasing dietary potassium and consumption of fruits, vegetables, and low-fat dairy, using the Dietary Approaches to Stop Hypertension (DASH) diet
- Smoking cessation
- Limit excessive alcohol intake (≤2 servings per day for men, ≤1 serving per day for women; one serving equivalent to 15 g ethanol)
- Exercise (walking, biking, swimming, etc., at least 30 minutes 3–4 times per week)
- Caffeine cessation
- Stress reduction
- Lifestyle modification for 4–8 weeks; if BP goal of <140/90 mmHg is not met, go to **B**.

B. First-line drug(s) for pharmacological treatment (ACE inhibitors or ARBs)

1. Start patient on benazepril (an ACE inhibitor) 10 mg once daily.
2. Measure K^+ and check BP 4 weeks after each change of benazepril dose.
3. If K^+ is 5.4 mEq/L or higher, decrease to previous dose.
4. If BP goal of <140/90 mmHg is not met at the 4-week follow-up visit, increase benazepril to 10 mg b.i.d.
5. Measure K^+ and recheck BP 4 weeks after dose increase; if K^+ is 5.4 mEq/L or higher, decrease to previous dose.
6. If BP goal of <140/90 mmHg is not met at the 4-week follow-up visit, increase benazepril to 20 mg b.i.d. (40 mg total, our maximum anti-hypertension dose).
7. Measure K^+ and recheck BP 4 weeks after dose increase; if K^+ is 5.4 mEq/L or higher, decrease to previous dose.
8. If the BP goal of <140/90 mmHg is not met at the 4-week follow-up visit after the maximal dose of an ACE inhibitor is prescribed, go to second-line drug (**C**).
9. If patient complains of a cough or angioedema (two other side effects in addition to hyperkalemia), discontinue benazepril and start losartan (Cozaar), an ARB, using a dose equivalency from Table 5.2.
10. If BP not at goal of <140/90 mmHg 4 weeks after the switch is made, increase losartan to maximal dose stepwise as described for benazepril, until goal is met.
11. Because ARBs can also raise K^+ levels, they cannot be substituted for an ACE inhibitor if the latter causes hyperkalemia.

Table 5.2. Benazepril-Losartan Dose Equivalency

ACE inhibitor	ARB
Benazepril 10 mg	Losartan 25 mg
Benazepril 20 mg	Losartan 50 mg
Benazepril 40 mg	Losartan 100 mg

12. If the BP goal of <140/90 mmHg is not met at the 4-week follow-up visit after the maximal dose of an ARB is prescribed, go to second-line drug (**C**).
13. If the dose of ACE inhibitor or ARB has to be decreased because of hyperkalemia, the BP goal will probably not be reached; in that case, maintain dose of ACE inhibitor or ARB not causing hyperkalemia and proceed to second-line drug (**C**).

C. Second-line drug (diuretic): Hydrochlorothiazide (HCTZ) (if eGFR is ≥30 mL/min) or indapamide (Lozol, if eGFR is <30 mL/min; in our experience, indapamide is a more effective and better tolerated choice than loop diuretics). To be used if BP goal of <140/90 mmHg is not achieved with a maximum (tolerated) dose of an ACE inhibitor or ARB.

1. If eGFR is ≥30 mL/min, add HCTZ 12.5 mg once daily, in the morning.
2. If BP goal of <140/90 mmHg is not met at the 4-week follow-up visit, increase HCTZ to 25 mg once daily in the morning (maximal dose).
3. If BP goal of <140/90 mmHg is not met at the 4-week follow-up visit, go to third-line drug (**D**).
4. If the eGFR is <30 mL/min, start indapamide 1.25 mg once daily, in the morning.
5. If BP goal of <140/90 mmHg is not met at the 4-week follow-up visit, increase indapamide dose to 2.5 mg once daily in the morning (maximal dose).
6. If BP goal of <140/90 mmHg is not met at the 4-week follow-up visit, go to third-line drug (**D**).

D. Third-line drug (NDHP CCB): Diltiazem (Cardizem) or verapamil (Calan). This drug is to be used if BP goal of <140/90 mmHg is not achieved with combination of maximal doses of the first- and second-line drugs.

1. Add extended-release diltiazem 180 mg once daily, in the evening.
2. If the BP goal of <140/90 mmHg is not met at the 4-week follow-up visit, increase to 180 mg b.i.d. (maximal dose).
3. If BP goal of <140/90 mmHg is not met at the 4-week follow-up visit and the patient is at the maximum dose of a combination of the first-, second-, and third-line drugs, go to fourth-line drug (**E**).

E. Fourth-line drug (direct vasodilators): Hydralazine. To be used if BP goal of <140/90 mmHg is not achieved with a combination of maximal doses of first-, second-, and third-line drugs.

1. Add hydralazine 50 mg b.i.d.
2. If BP goal of <140/90 mmHg is not met at 4-week follow-up visit, increase to 100 mg b.i.d. (maximal dose).
3. If BP goal of <140/90 mmHg is not met at 4-week follow-up visit *and* patient is taking maximal doses of four classes of drugs (ACE inhibitor or ARB, diuretic, NDHP CCB, and direct vasodilator), consider referral to a hypertension expert (e.g., a nephrologist).

REFERENCES

1. Lewington S, Clarke R, Qizilbash N, et al. Age-specific relevance of usual blood pressure to vascular mortality: a meta-analysis of individual data for one million adults in 61 prospective studies. *Lancet* 2002;360:1903–1913

2. Curb JD, Pressel SL, Cutler JA, et al.; Systolic Hypertension in the Elderly Program Cooperative Research Group. Effect of diuretic-based antihypertensive treatment on cardiovascular disease risk in older diabetic patients with isolated systolic hypertension. *JAMA* 1996;276:1886–1892

3. UK Prospective Diabetes Study Group. Tight blood pressure control and risk of macrovascular and microvascular complications in type 2 diabetes: UKPDS 38. *BMJ* 1998;317:703–713

4. Hansson L, Zanchetti A, Carruthers SG, et al.; HOT Study Group. Effects of intensive blood-pressure lowering and low-dose aspirin in patients with hypertension: principal results of the Hypertension Optimal Treatment (HOT) randomised trial. *Lancet* 1998;351:1755–1762

5. Tuomilehto J, Rastenyte D, Birkenhager WH, et al.; Systolic Hypertension in Europe Trial Investigators. Effects of calcium-channel blockade in older patients with diabetes and systolic hypertension. *N Engl J Med* 1999;340:677–684

6. Estacio RO, Jeffers BW, Gifford N, Schrier RW. Effect of blood pressure control on diabetic microvascular complications in patients with hypertension and type 2 diabetes. *Diabetes Care* 2000;23(Suppl. 2):B54–B64

7. Patel A, MacMahon S, Chalmers J, et al. Effects of a fixed combination of perindopril and indapamide on macrovascular and microvascular outcomes in patients with type 2 diabetes mellitus (the ADVANCE trial): a randomised controlled trial. *Lancet* 2007;370:829–840

8. Cushman WC, Evans GW, Byington RP, et al. Effects of intensive blood-pressure control in type 2 diabetes mellitus. *N Engl J Med* 2010;362:1575–1585

9. McBrien K, Rabi DM, Campbell N, et al. Intensive and standard blood pressure targets in patients with type 2 diabetes mellitus: systematic review and meta-analysis. *Arch Intern Med* 2012;172:1296–1303

10. Arguedas JA, Leiva V, Wright JM. Blood pressure targets for hypertension in people with diabetes mellitus. *Cochrane Database Syst Rev* 2013;10:CD008277

11. Parving HH, Andersen AR, Smidt UM, et al. Effect of antihypertensive treatment on kidney function in diabetic nephropathy. *Br Med J (Clin Res Ed)* 1987;294:1443–1447

12. Bakris GL. Progression of diabetic nephropathy: a focus on arterial pressure level and methods of reduction. *Diabetes Res Clin Pract* 1998;39(Suppl.):S35–S42

13. Leske MC, Wu SY, Hennis A, et al. Hyperglycemia, blood pressure, and the 9-year incidence of diabetic retinopathy: the Barbados Eye Studies. *Ophthalmology* 2005;112:799–805

14. Chew EY, Ambrosius WT, Davis MD, et al. Effects of medical therapies on retinopathy progression in type 2 diabetes. *N Engl J Med* 2010;363:233–244

15. Pickering TG, Hall JE, Appel LJ, et al. Recommendations for blood pressure measurement in humans and experimental animals: part 1: blood pressure measurement in humans: a statement for professionals from the Subcommittee of Professional and Public Education of the American Heart Association Council on High Blood Pressure Research. *Circulation* 2005;111:697–716

16. American Diabetes Association. Cardiovascular disease and risk management. *Diabetes Care* 2016;39(Suppl. 1):S60–S71

17. Wright JT Jr, Williamson JD, Whelton PK, et al. A randomized trial of intensive versus standard blood-pressure control. *N Engl J Med* 2015;373:2103–2116

18. Brunstrom M, Carlberg B. Effect of antihypertensive treatment at different blood pressure levels in patients with diabetes mellitus: systematic review and meta-analyses. *BMJ* 2016;352:i717

19. Sacks FM, Svetkey LP, Vollmer WM, et al.; DASH-Sodium Collaborative Research Group. Effects on blood pressure of reduced dietary sodium and the Dietary Approaches to Stop Hypertension (DASH) diet. *N Engl J Med* 2001;344:3–10

20. Bray GA, Vollmer WM, Sacks FM, et al. A further subgroup analysis of the effects of the DASH diet and three dietary sodium levels on blood pressure: results of the DASH-Sodium Trial. *Am J Cardiol* 2004;94:222–227

21. American Diabetes Association. Foundations of care and comprehensive medical evaluation. *Diabetes Care* 2016;39(Suppl. 1):S23–S35

22. Maillot M, Drewnowski A. A conflict between nutritionally adequate diets and meeting the 2010 dietary guidelines for sodium. *Am J Prev Med* 2012;42:174–179

23. Thomas MC, Moran J, Forsblom C, et al. The association between dietary sodium intake, ESRD, and all-cause mortality in patients with type 1 diabetes. *Diabetes Care* 2011;34:861–866

24. Ekinci EI, Clarke S, Thomas MC, et al. Dietary salt intake and mortality in patients with type 2 diabetes. *Diabetes Care* 2011;34:703–709

25. Azadbakht L, Fard NR, Karimi M, et al. Effects of the Dietary Approaches to Stop Hypertension (DASH) eating plan on cardiovascular risks among type 2 diabetic patients: a randomized crossover clinical trial. *Diabetes Care* 2011;34:55–57

26. Cornelissen VA, Smart NA. Exercise training for blood pressure: a systematic review and meta-analysis. *J Am Heart Assoc* 2013;2:e004473

27. Colberg SR, Sigal RJ, Fernhall B, et al. Exercise and type 2 diabetes: the American College of Sports Medicine and the American Diabetes Association: joint position statement. *Diabetes Care* 2010;33:e147–e167

28. Wald DS, Law M, Morris JK, et al. Combination therapy versus monotherapy in reducing blood pressure: meta-analysis on 11,000 participants from 42 trials. *Am J Med* 2009;122:290–300

29. Turnbull F. Effects of different blood-pressure-lowering regimens on major cardiovascular events: results of prospectively-designed overviews of randomised trials. *Lancet* 2003;362:1527–1535

30. ALLHAT Collaborative Research Group. Major cardiovascular events in hypertensive patients randomized to doxazosin vs chlorthalidone: the antihypertensive and lipid-lowering treatment to prevent heart attack trial (ALLHAT). *JAMA* 2000;283:1967–1975

31. Vejakama P, Thakkinstian A, Lertrattananon D, et al. Reno-protective effects of renin-angiotensin system blockade in type 2 diabetic patients: a systematic review and network meta-analysis. *Diabetologia* 2012;55:566–578

32. Wu HY, Huang JW, Lin HJ, et al. Comparative effectiveness of renin-angiotensin system blockers and other antihypertensive drugs in patients with diabetes: systematic review and bayesian network meta-analysis. *BMJ* 2013;347:f6008

33. Zhao P, Xu P, Wan C, Wang Z. Evening versus morning dosing regimen drug therapy for hypertension. *Cochrane Database Syst Rev* 2011:CD004184

34. Hermida RC, Ayala DE, Mojon A, Fernandez JR. Influence of time of day of blood pressure-lowering treatment on cardiovascular risk in hypertensive patients with type 2 diabetes. *Diabetes Care* 2011;34:1270–1276

35. Macias Heras M, del Castillo Rodriguez N, Navarro Gonzalez JF. The renin-angiotensin-aldosterone system in renal and cardiovascular disease and the effects of its pharmacological blockade. *J Diabetes Metab* 2012;3:171

36. Brown NJ, Vaughan DE. Angiotensin-converting enzyme inhibitors. *Circulation* 1998;97:1411–1420

37. Cheng J, Zhang W, Zhang X, et al. Effect of angiotensin-converting enzyme inhibitors and angiotensin II receptor blockers on all-cause mortality, cardiovascular deaths, and cardiovascular events in patients with diabetes mellitus: a meta-analysis. *JAMA Intern Med* 2014;174:773–785

38. van Vark LC, Bertrand M, Akkerhuis KM, et al. Angiotensin-converting enzyme inhibitors reduce mortality in hypertension: a meta-analysis of randomized clinical trials of renin-angiotensin-aldosterone system inhibitors involving 158,998 patients. *Eur Heart J* 2012;33:2088–2097

39. Peck RN, Smart LR, Beier R, et al. Difference in blood pressure response to ACE-inhibitor monotherapy between black and white adults with arterial hypertension: a meta-analysis of 13 clinical trials. *BMC Nephrol* 2013;14:201

40. Flack JM, Sica DA, Bakris G, et al. Management of high blood pressure in blacks: an update of the International Society on Hypertension in Blacks consensus statement. *Hypertension* 2010;56:780–800

41. Taylor AA, Siragy H, Nesbitt S. Angiotensin receptor blockers: pharmacology, efficacy, and safety. *J Clin Hypertens (Greenwich)* 2011;13:677–686

42. Akioyamen L, Levine M, Sherifali D, et al. Cardiovascular and cerebrovascular outcomes of long-term angiotensin receptor blockade: meta-analyses of trials in essential hypertension. *J Am Soc Hypertens* 2016;10:55–69 e51

43. Dusing R, Sellers F. ACE inhibitors, angiotensin receptor blockers and direct renin inhibitors in combination: a review of their role after the ONTARGET trial. *Curr Med Res Opin* 2009;25:2287–2301

44. Duarte JD, Cooper-DeHoff RM. Mechanisms for blood pressure lowering and metabolic effects of thiazide and thiazide-like diuretics. *Expert Rev Cardiovasc Ther* 2010;8:793–802

45. Horita S, Seki G, Yamada H, Suzuki M, Koike K, Fujita T. Insulin resistance, obesity, hypertension, and renal sodium transport. *Int J Hypertens* 2011;2011:391762

46. ALLHAT Officers and Coordinators for the ALLHAT Collaborative Research Group. Major outcomes in high-risk hypertensive patients randomized to angiotensin-converting enzyme inhibitor or calcium channel blocker vs diuretic: the Antihypertensive and Lipid-Lowering Treatment to Prevent Heart Attack Trial (ALLHAT). *JAMA* 2002;288:2981–2997

47. Chobanian AV, Bakris GL, Black HR, et al. The seventh report of the Joint National Committee on Prevention, Detection, Evaluation, and Treatment of High Blood Pressure: the JNC 7 report. *JAMA* 2003;289:2560–2572

48. James PA, Oparil S, Carter BL, et al. 2014 Evidence-based guideline for the management of high blood pressure in adults: report from the panel members appointed to the Eighth Joint National Committee (JNC 8). *JAMA* 2014;311:507–520

49. Carter BL, Einhorn PT, Brands M, et al. Thiazide-induced dysglycemia: call for research from a working group from the National Heart, Lung, and Blood Institute. *Hypertension* 2008;52:30–36

50. Ernst ME, Moser M. Use of diuretics in patients with hypertension. *N Engl J Med* 2009;361:2153–2164

51. Wermers RA, Kearns AE, Jenkins GD, Melton LJ 3rd. Incidence and clinical spectrum of thiazide-associated hypercalcemia. *Am J Med* 2007;120:911 e9–15

52. Kasiske BL, Ma JZ, Kalil RS, Louis TA. Effects of antihypertensive therapy on serum lipids. *Ann Intern Med* 1995;122:133–141

53. Malha L, Mann SJ. Loop diuretics in the treatment of hypertension. *Curr Hypertens Rep* 2016;18:27

54. Musini VM, Rezapour P, Wright JM, Bassett K, Jauca CD. Blood pressure lowering efficacy of loop diuretics for primary hypertension. *Cochrane Database Syst Rev* 2012:CD003825

55. Sica DA. Pharmacotherapy review: calcium channel blockers. *J Clin Hypertens (Greenwich)* 2006;8:53–56

56. Tatti P, Pahor M, Byington RP, et al. Outcome results of the Fosinopril Versus Amlodipine Cardiovascular Events Randomized Trial (FACET) in patients with hypertension and NIDDM. *Diabetes Care* 1998;21:597–603

57. Estacio RO, Jeffers BW, Hiatt WR, et al. The effect of nisoldipine as compared with enalapril on cardiovascular outcomes in patients with non-insulin-dependent diabetes and hypertension. *N Engl J Med* 1998;338:645–652

58. Opie LH, Schall R. Evidence-based evaluation of calcium channel blockers for hypertension: equality of mortality and cardiovascular risk relative to conventional therapy. *J Am Coll Cardiol* 2002;39:315–322

59. Jeffers BW, Robbins J, Bhambri R, Wajsbrot D. A systematic review on the efficacy of amlodipine in the treatment of patients with hypertension with concomitant diabetes mellitus and/or renal dysfunction, when compared with other classes of antihypertensive medication. *Am J Ther* 2015;22:322–341

60. Pahor M, Psaty BM, Alderman MH, et al. Health outcomes associated with calcium antagonists compared with other first-line antihypertensive therapies: a meta-analysis of randomised controlled trials. *Lancet* 2000;356:1949–1954

61. Chen N, Zhou M, Yang M, et al. Calcium channel blockers versus other classes of drugs for hypertension. *Cochrane Database Syst Rev* 2010:CD003654

62. Chen GJ, Yang MS. The effects of calcium channel blockers in the prevention of stroke in adults with hypertension: a meta-analysis of data from 273,543 participants in 31 randomized controlled trials. *PLoS One* 2013;8:e57854

63. Brewster LM, van Montfrans GA, Kleijnen J. Systematic review: antihypertensive drug therapy in black patients. *Ann Intern Med* 2004;141:614–627

64. Nguyen TT, Kaufman JS, Whitsel EA, Cooper RS. Racial differences in blood pressure response to calcium channel blocker monotherapy: a meta-analysis. *Am J Hypertens* 2009;22:911–917

65. Leenen FH, Nwachuku CE, Black HR, et al. Clinical events in high-risk hypertensive patients randomly assigned to calcium channel blocker versus angiotensin-converting enzyme inhibitor in the Antihypertensive and Lipid-Lowering Treatment to Prevent Heart Attack Trial. *Hypertension* 2006;48:374–384

66. Melbourne Diabetic Nephropathy Study Group. Comparison between perindopril and nifedipine in hypertensive and normotensive diabetic patients with microalbuminuria. *BMJ* 1991;302:210–216

67. Velussi M, Brocco E, Frigato F, et al. Effects of cilazapril and amlodipine on kidney function in hypertensive NIDDM patients. *Diabetes* 1996;45:216–222

68. Chan JC, Cockram CS, Nicholls MG, et al. Comparison of enalapril and nifedipine in treating non-insulin dependent diabetes associated with hypertension: one year analysis. *BMJ* 1992;305:981–985

69. Chan JC, Ko GT, Leung DH, et al. Long-term effects of angiotensin-converting enzyme inhibition and metabolic control in hypertensive type 2 diabetic patients. *Kidney Int* 2000;57:590–600

70. Tarif N, Bakris GL. Preservation of renal function: the spectrum of effects by calcium-channel blockers. *Nephrol Dial Transplant* 1997;12:2244–2250

71. Smith AC, Toto R, Bakris GL. Differential effects of calcium channel blockers on size selectivity of proteinuria in diabetic glomerulopathy. *Kidney Int* 1998;54:889–896

72. Toto RD, Tian M, Fakouhi K, Champion A, Bacher P. Effects of calcium channel blockers on proteinuria in patients with diabetic nephropathy. *J Clin Hypertens (Greenwich)* 2008;10:761–769

73. Clark DW. Genetically determined variability in acetylation and oxidation: therapeutic implications. *Drugs* 1985;29:342–375

74. Sica DA. Minoxidil: an underused vasodilator for resistant or severe hypertension. *J Clin Hypertens (Greenwich)* 2004;6:283–287

75. Gottlieb SS, McCarter RJ, Vogel RA. Effect of beta-blockade on mortality among high-risk and low-risk patients after myocardial infarction. *N Engl J Med* 1998;339:489–497

76. Freemantle N, Cleland J, Young P, Mason J, Harrison J. β Blockade after myocardial infarction: systematic review and meta regression analysis. *BMJ* 1999;318:1730–1737

77. Bangalore S, Messerli FH, Kostis JB, Pepine CJ. Cardiovascular protection using beta-blockers: a critical review of the evidence. *J Am Coll Cardiol* 2007;50:563–572

78. Bell DS, Lukas MA, Holdbrook FK, Fowler MB. The effect of carvedilol on mortality risk in heart failure patients with diabetes: results of a meta-analysis. *Curr Med Res Opin* 2006;22:287–296

79. Cruickshank JM. Beta-blockers and diabetes: the bad guys come good. *Cardiovasc Drugs Ther* 2002;16:457–470

80. UK Prospective Diabetes Study Group. Efficacy of atenolol and captopril in reducing risk of macrovascular and microvascular complications in type 2 diabetes: UKPDS 39. *BMJ* 1998;317:713–720

81. Lindholm LH, Ibsen H, Dahlof B, et al. Cardiovascular morbidity and mortality in patients with diabetes in the Losartan Intervention For Endpoint reduction in hypertension study (LIFE): a randomised trial against atenolol. *Lancet* 2002;359:1004–1010

82. DiNicolantonio JJ, Fares H, Niazi AK, et al. β-Blockers in hypertension, diabetes, heart failure and acute myocardial infarction: a review of the literature. *Open Heart* 2015;2:e000230

83. Aberg H, Morlin C, Lithell H; EGTA Group. Different long-term metabolic effects of enalapril and atenolol in patients with mild hypertension. *J Hum Hypertens* 1995;9:149–153

84. Jacob S, Klimm HJ, Rett K, et al. Effects of moxonidine vs. metoprolol on blood pressure and metabolic control in hypertensive subjects with type 2 diabetes. *Exp Clin Endocrinol Diabetes* 2004;112:315–322

85. Pischon T, Sharma AM. Use of beta-blockers in obesity hypertension: potential role of weight gain. *Obes Rev* 2001;2:275–280

86. Bakris GL, Fonseca V, Katholi RE, et al. Metabolic effects of carvedilol vs metoprolol in patients with type 2 diabetes mellitus and hypertension: a randomized controlled trial. *JAMA* 2004;292:2227–2236

87. Messerli FH, Bell DS, Fonseca V, et al. Body weight changes with beta-blocker use: results from GEMINI. *Am J Med* 2007;120:610–615

88. Fonseca VA. Effects of beta-blockers on glucose and lipid metabolism. *Curr Med Res Opin* 2010;26:615–629

89. Vidt DG. Mechanism of action, pharmacokinetics, adverse effects, and therapeutic uses of amiloride hydrochloride, a new potassium-sparing diuretic. *Pharmacotherapy* 1981;1:179–187

90. Pitt B, Zannad F, Remme WJ, et al.; Randomized Aldactone Evaluation Study Investigators. The effect of spironolactone on morbidity and mortality in patients with severe heart failure. *N Engl J Med* 1999;341:709–717

91. Maron BA, Leopold JA. Aldosterone receptor antagonists: effective but often forgotten. *Circulation* 2010;121:934–939

92. Pitt B, Remme W, Zannad F, et al. Eplerenone, a selective aldosterone blocker, in patients with left ventricular dysfunction after myocardial infarction. *N Engl J Med* 2003;348:1309–1321

93. Navaneethan SD, Nigwekar SU, Sehgal AR, Strippoli GF. Aldosterone antagonists for preventing the progression of chronic kidney disease: a systematic review and meta-analysis. *Clin J Am Soc Nephrol* 2009;4:542–551

94. Takahashi S, Katada J, Daida H, et al. Effects of mineralocorticoid receptor antagonists in patients with hypertension and diabetes mellitus: a systematic review and meta-analysis. *J Hum Hypertension* 2016;30:534–542

95. Sen S, Sabirli S, Ozyigit T, Uresin Y. Aliskiren: review of efficacy and safety data with focus on past and recent clinical trials. *Ther Adv Chronic Dis* 2013;4:232–241

96. Parving HH, Persson F, Lewis JB, et al. Aliskiren combined with losartan in type 2 diabetes and nephropathy. *N Engl J Med* 2008;358:2433–2446

97. Parving HH, Brenner BM, McMurray JJ, et al. Cardiorenal end points in a trial of aliskiren for type 2 diabetes. *N Engl J Med* 2012;367:2204–2213

98. Vongpatanasin W, Kario K, Atlas SA, Victor RG. Central sympatholytic drugs. *J Clin Hypertens (Greenwich)* 2011;13:658–661

99. Shamon SD, Perez MI. Blood pressure lowering efficacy of reserpine for primary hypertension. *Cochrane Database Syst Rev* 2009:CD007655

100. Lepor H. Alpha blockers for the treatment of benign prostatic hyperplasia. *Rev Urol* 2007;9:181–190

101. Heran BS, Galm BP, Wright JM. Blood pressure lowering efficacy of alpha blockers for primary hypertension. *Cochrane Database Syst Rev* 2012:CD004643

Appendix

ENGLISH

Instructions for Overweight or Obese Patients

- Insulins: NPH (Humulin N, Novolin N) taken before supper or bedtime

- Insulins: Glargine (Lantus, Tuojeo, Basaglar), Detemir (Levemir), or Degludec (Tresiba) taken before bedtime:
  - Test blood glucose daily before breakfast.
  - Every morning the result is greater than 130 mg/dL, increase the insulin dose by 2 units that evening. (If you are taking NPH insulin before breakfast, do not change that dose.)
  - Every morning the result is less than 70 mg/dL, decrease the insulin dose by 2 units that evening. (If you are taking NPH insulin before breakfast, do not change that dose.)
  - If there have been no changes in the insulin dose for 1 week, do not change the dose anymore.

- Insulins: Glargine (Lantus, Tuojeo, Basaglar), Detemir (Levemir), or Degludec (Tresiba) taken before breakfast:
  - Test blood glucose daily before breakfast.
  - Every morning the result is greater than 130 mg/dL, increase the insulin dose that morning by 2 units.
  - Every morning the result is less than 70 mg/dL, decrease the insulin dose that morning by 2 units.
  - If there have been no changes in the insulin dose for 1 week, do not change the dose anymore.

- Insulins: Glargine (Lantus, Tuojeo, Basaglar), Detemir (Levemir), or Degludec (Tresiba) taken before breakfast AND before bedtime:
  - Test blood glucose daily before breakfast.
  - Every morning the result is greater than 130 mg/dL, increase BOTH the morning AND bedtime insulin doses by 2 units each.
  - Every morning that the result is less than 70 mg/dL, decrease BOTH the morning AND bedtime insulin doses by 2 units each.
  - If there have been no changes in the insulin doses for 1 week, do not change them anymore.

151

Instructions for Lean Patients

- Insulins: NPH (Humulin N, Novolin N) taken before supper or bedtime
- Insulins: Glargine (Lantus, Tuojeo, Basaglar), Detemir (Levemir), or Degludec (Tresiba) taken before bedtime:
  - Test blood glucose daily before breakfast.
  - Every morning the result is greater than 130 mg/dL, increase the insulin dose by 1 unit that evening. (If you are taking NPH insulin before breakfast, do not change that dose.)
  - Every morning the result is less than 70 mg/dL, decrease the insulin dose by 1 unit that evening. (If you are taking NPH insulin before breakfast, do not change that dose.)
  - If there have been no changes in the insulin dose for 1 week, do not change it anymore.

- Insulins: Glargine (Lantus, Tuojeo, Basaglar), Detemir (Levemir), or Degludec (Tresiba) taken before breakfast:
  - Test blood glucose daily before breakfast.
  - Every morning the result is greater than 130 mg/dL, increase the insulin dose that morning by 1 unit.
  - Every morning the result is less than 70 mg/dL, decrease the insulin dose that morning by 1 unit.
  - If there have been no changes in the insulin dose for 1 week, do not change them anymore.

- Insulins: Glargine (Lantus, Tuojeo, Basaglar), Detemir (Levemir), or Degludec (Tresiba) taken before breakfast AND before bedtime:
  - Test blood glucose daily before breakfast.
  - Every morning the result is greater than 130 mg/dL, increase BOTH the morning AND bedtime insulin doses by 1 unit each.
  - Every morning the result is less than 70 mg/dL, decrease BOTH the morning AND bedtime insulin doses by 1 unit each.
  - If there have been no changes in the insulin doses for 1 week, do not change them anymore.

ESPAÑOL

Instrucciones para pacientes con sobrepeso u obesos

- Insulinas: NPH (Humulin N, Novolin N) que se pone antes de la cena o antes de irse a dormir

- Insulinas: Glargina (Lantus, Tuojeo, Basaglar), Detemir (Levemir) o Degludec (Tresiba) que se pone antes de irse a dormir:
  - Hágase la prueba de glucosa en la sangre todos los días antes del desayuno.
  - Cada mañana que su nivel de glucosa es mayor de 130 mg/dL, aumente la dosis de insulina que se pondrá en la noche en 2 unidades. (Si usted está usando insulina NPH antes del desayuno, no cambie la dosis).
  - Cada mañana que su nivel de glucosa es menos de 70 mg/dL, disminuya la dosis de insulina que se pondrá en la noche en 2 unidades. (Si usted está usando insulina NPH antes del desayuno, no cambie la dosis).
  - Si no ha habido cambios en la dosis de insulina durante 1 semana, ya no vuelva a cambiar la dosis.

- Insulinas: Glargina (Lantus, Tuojeo, Basaglar), Detemir (Levemir) o Degludec (Tresiba) que se pone antes del desayuno:
  - Hágase la prueba de glucosa en la sangre todos los días antes del desayuno.
  - Cada mañana que su nivel de glucosa es mayor de 130 mg/dL, aumente la dosis de insulina esa mañana en 2 unidades.
  - Cada mañana que su nivel de glucosa es menos de 70 mg/dL, disminuya la dosis de insulina esa mañana en 2 unidades.
  - Si no ha habido cambios en la dosis de insulina durante 1 semana, ya no vuelva a cambiar la dosis.

- Insulinas: Glargina (Lantus, Tuojeo, Basaglar), Detemir (Levemir) o Degludec (Tresiba) que se pone antes del desayuno Y antes de irse a dormir:
  - Hágase la prueba de glucosa en la sangre todos los días antes del desayuno.
  - Cada mañana que su nivel de glucosa es mayor de 130 mg/dL, aumente AMBAS DOSIS, la insulina de la mañana Y la insulina antes de dormir en 2 unidades adicionales cada una.
  - Cada mañana que su nivel de glucosa es menos de 70 mg/dL, disminuya AMBAS DOSIS, la insulina de la mañana Y la insulina antes de dormir en 2 unidades menos cada una.
  - Si no ha habido cambios en las dosis de insulina durante 1 semana, ya no vuelva a cambiar la dosis.

Instrucciones para pacientes delgados

- Insulinas: NPH (Humulin N, Novolin N) que se pone antes de la cena o antes de irse a dormir

- Insulinas: Glargina (Lantus, Tuojeo, Basaglar), Detemir (Levemir) o Degludec (Tresiba) que se pone antes de irse a dormir:
  - Hágase la prueba de glucosa en la sangre todos los días antes del desayuno.
  - Cada mañana que su nivel de glucosa es mayor de 130 mg/dL, aumente la dosis de insulina que se pondrá en la noche en 1 unidad. (Si usted está usando insulina NPH antes del desayuno, no cambie esa dosis).
  - Cada mañana que su nivel de glucosa es menos de 70 mg/dL, disminuya la dosis de insulina que se pondrá en la noche en 1 unidad. (Si usted está usando insulina NPH antes del desayuno, no cambie esa dosis).
  - Si no ha habido cambios en la dosis de insulina durante 1 semana, ya no vuelva a cambiar la dosis.

- Insulinas: Glargina (Lantus, Tuojeo, Basaglar), Detemir (Levemir) o Degludec (Tresiba) que se pone antes del desayuno:
  - Hágase la prueba de glucosa en la sangre todos los días antes del desayuno.
  - Cada mañana que su nivel de glucosa es mayor de 130 mg/dL, aumente la dosis de insulina esa mañana en 1 unidad.
  - Cada mañana que su nivel de glucosa es menos de 70 mg/dL, disminuya la dosis de insulina esa mañana en 1 unidad.
  - Si no ha habido cambios en la dosis de insulina durante 1 semana, ya no vuelva a cambiar la dosis.

- Insulinas: Glargina (Lantus, Tuojeo, Basaglar), Detemir (Levemir) o Degludec (Tresiba) que se pone antes del desayuno Y antes de irse a dormir:
  - Hágase la prueba de glucosa en la sangre todos los días antes del desayuno.
  - Cada mañana que su nivel de glucosa es mayor de 130 mg/dL, aumente AMBAS DOSIS, la insulina de la mañana Y la insulina antes de dormir en 1 unidad adicional cada una.
  - Cada mañana que su nivel de glucosa es menos de 70 mg/dL, disminuya AMBAS DOSIS, la insulina de la mañana Y la insulina antes de dormir en 1 unidad menos cada una.
  - Si no ha habido cambios en las dosis de insulina durante 1 semana, ya no vuelva a cambiar la dosis.

Index

CPSIA information can be obtained
at www.ICGtesting.com
Printed in the USA
FFOW05n0955150317

9 781580 406017